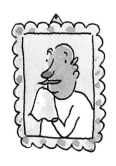

Health And Healing
The Natural Way

FIGHTING
ALLERGIES

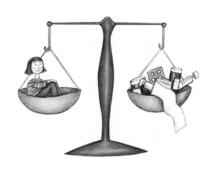

HEALTH AND HEALING
THE NATURAL WAY

FIGHTING ALLERGIES

PUBLISHED BY

THE READER'S DIGEST ASSOCIATION LIMITED

LONDON NEW YORK SYDNEY MONTREAL

FIGHTING ALLERGIES
was created and produced by
Carroll & Brown Limited
20 Lonsdale Road, London NW6 6RD
for The Reader's Digest Association Limited, London

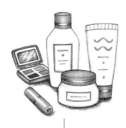

CARROLL & BROWN

Publishing Director Denis Kennedy
Art Director Chrissie Lloyd

Managing Editor Sandra Rigby
Managing Art Editor Tracy Timson

Editor Joel Levy

Art Editor Simon Daley
Designer Evie Loizides

Photographers David Murray, Jules Selmes

Production Wendy Rogers, Clair Reynolds

Computer Management John Clifford, Karen Kloot

First English Edition Copyright © 1998
The Reader's Digest Association Limited,
11 Westferry Circus, Canary Wharf,
London E14 4HE

Copyright © 1998
The Reader's Digest Association Far East Limited
Philippines Copyright © 1998
The Reader's Digest Association Far East Limited

Reprinted 2001

ISBN 0 276 42268 6

Reproduced by Colourscan, Singapore
Printing and binding: Printer Industria Gráfica S.A., Barcelona

CONSULTANTS

Dr Honor M. Anthony MB ChB
Specialist in Environmental Medicine, Leeds

Roger Newman Turner BAc, ND, DO
Member of the Register of Naturopaths
Member of the Register of Osteopaths

CONTRIBUTORS

Dr Paul J. August FRCP
Consultant Dermatologist

Dr Keith K. Eaton LRCPE, LRCSE, LRFPSG
Consultant Allergist, Princess Margaret Hospital, Windsor

Dr David L.J. Freed MB, ChB, MD, CBiol, MIBiol
Consulting Allergist, Salford Allergy Clinic

Dr D. Jonathan Maberly FRCP, FRACP
Consultant Physician
Medical Director of the Airedale Allergy Centre

Dr John R. Mansfield LRCP, MRCS, DRCOG
Consultant Allergist, Burghwood Clinic

Dr Michael J. Radcliffe MB, ChB, MRCGP, FAAEM
Associate Specialist in Allergy, Middlesex Hospital

Dr Michael A. Tettenborn MB, FRCP, FRCPCH
Consultant in Paediatrics and Child Health,
North Downs NHS Trust

Dr Richard Turner MB, MRCP
Specialist in Allergy, North Hampshire Hospital, Basingstoke

FOR READER'S DIGEST

Series Editor Christine Noble
Editorial Assistant Caroline Boucher

READER'S DIGEST GENERAL BOOKS

Editorial Director Cortina Butler
Art Director Nick Clark

The information in this book is for reference only;
it is not intended as a substitute for a doctor's diagnosis and care.
The editors urge anyone with continuing medical problems
or symptoms to consult a doctor.

FIGHTING ALLERGIES

More and more people today are choosing to take greater responsibility for their own health rather than relying on the doctor to step in with a cure when something goes wrong. We now recognise that we can influence our health by making an improvement in lifestyle – a better diet, more exercise and reduced stress. People are also becoming increasingly aware that there are other healing methods – some new, others very ancient – that can help to prevent illness or be used as a complement to orthodox medicine.

The series *Health and Healing the Natural Way* will help you to make your own health choices by giving you clear, comprehensive, straightforward and encouraging information and advice about methods of improving your health. The series explains the many different natural therapies now available – aromatherapy, herbalism, acupressure and many others – and the circumstances in which they may be of benefit when used in conjunction with conventional medicine.

FIGHTING ALLERGIES introduces the complex and often controversial subject of allergies. Some of those working in this field regard allergies as the next major health issue in the developed world, but for the millions suffering today there is a surprising lack of support from mainstream medicine. *Fighting Allergies* presents both the conventional and complementary therapies available for the management of allergies, and also surveys the lifestyle, environmental and dietary issues that underlie the problems of allergy. It aims to provide the information you need to understand allergies, and explains how to detect and manage allergic conditions. More than this, it reveals the range of both everyday and serious illnesses which may be caused, either partly or entirely, by allergy, and highlights the complex interactions between diet, environment and lifestyle in general health.

CONTENTS

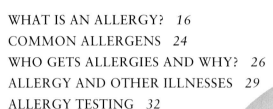

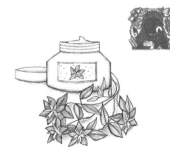

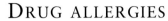

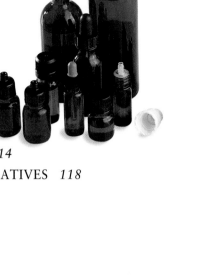

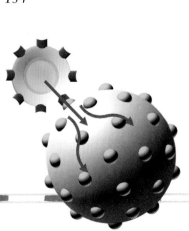

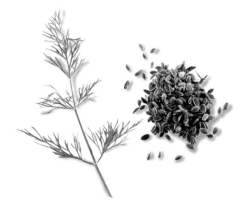

ALLERGY ALERT

There is evidence to suggest that allergies may be the major health issue of the next century. What steps can you take to protect yourself and your family?

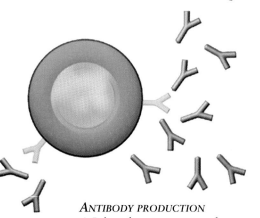

ANTIBODY PRODUCTION
A B-lymphocyte – a type of immune cell – acts as an antibody-producing 'factory', making the antibodies which can be the key players in allergic reactions.

EDWARD JENNER (1749–1823)
In 1796 this English physician developed the technique of vaccination against smallpox. Public demonstrations like the one shown below helped to convince the medical establishment of the value of his work.

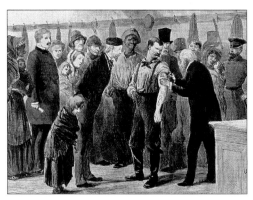

Allergies are often perceived as little more than a minor irritation. But as we near the turn of the century it is becoming increasingly apparent that well-known conditions such as hay fever and asthma may be just the tip of an allergy iceberg. There is considerable evidence that allergies could be causing or exacerbating a wide range of physical and mental disorders, but as yet this remains unrecognised by the mainstream medical fraternity. How can such an important health issue be so marginalised? The roots of the controversy stretch far back into medical history.

In 1906 a Viennese physician called Clemens von Pirquet coined the term allergy to describe how repeatedly vaccinated children developed an adverse immune reaction (serum sickness) to a substance which should have been harmless. Similar adverse reactions had previously been noted by the Romans, ancient Greeks and medieval Chinese, but von Pirquet put a name to the condition. What lay behind von Pirquet's discovery?

THE HISTORY OF ALLERGIES

In medieval times physicians observed that if a person recovered from the plague, he or she would subsequently be immune to it. Medieval philosophers in China developed a crude form of immunisation for smallpox, called variolation. The technique was introduced to Europe in the 18th century, but carried considerable risks and was soon supplanted by 'vaccination', a technique developed by the English doctor Edward Jenner.

It was not until the 19th and 20th centuries that scientific discoveries helped to uncover how this new technique was capable of conferring immunity to disease. It was found that the state of immunity was due, at least in part, to protein molecules in the blood called antibodies, and that the production of antibodies is caused by the presence of a foreign body or 'antigen' – normally a harmful substance such as a germ. However, it was also found that non-dangerous, non-infectious materials, like pollen or even foods, could give rise to antibody formation. Injecting a serum containing antibodies could be life-saving, but if a patient needed several injections of that serum over a few days or weeks, the result was the painful and sometimes life-threatening 'serum sickness'. Von Pirquet noticed this effect, and coined the term allergy to describe it.

Before long it became clear that the skin rashes which appeared on some people after eating strawberries or shellfish and the sneezing attacks caused by exposure to pollen also resulted from this changed reactivity, and doctors realised that these conditions were also caused by allergy.

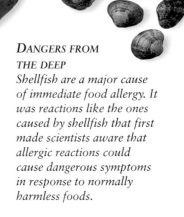

DANGERS FROM THE DEEP
Shellfish are a major cause of immediate food allergy. It was reactions like the ones caused by shellfish that first made scientists aware that allergic reactions could cause dangerous symptoms in response to normally harmless foods.

THE ROOTS OF CONTROVERSY

Now that allergies had been identified, scientists went to work on identifying the elements of the immune system that are involved, and the mechanisms that underlie allergic reactions. By the late 1960s the antibody responsible for classic allergic reactions such as hay fever and skin rashes was identified, and named immunoglobulin E (IgE, see Chapter 1). This discovery marked the movement of the discipline into an increasingly strict scientific mode, with demarcations between what is considered an allergy and what isn't.

As the scientific approach to allergies was becoming more rigid, some doctors were becoming increasingly aware that their clinical experience was at odds with conventional dogma. At the forefront of this group was Theron G. Randolph, MD, an American physician whose clinical observations led him to believe that at least 30 per cent of his patients were suffering from allergies. By paying careful attention to their diets and their working and living environments he was able to identify trigger substances that conventional allergy did not recognise, and, by reducing his patients' exposure to them, cure illnesses that conventional opinion did not even recognise as allergic disorders. Randolph founded the

IgE DISCOVERERS
In 1967, Teruko and Kimishige Ishizaka identified gamma E globulin, an antibody responsible for hay fever, eczema and asthma, which later became known as IgE. This discovery provided the basis for a more scientific bent to the study of allergies.

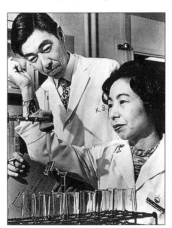

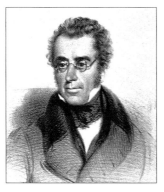

JOHN BOSTOCK
In the summer of 1819, John Bostock spoke to the Royal Medical Society of London of his 'periodical affection of the eyes and chest' which he referred to as 'summer catarrh'. The condition later became popularly known as hay fever.

A DEVELOPING PROBLEM
The modern lifestyle of the developed world may be at the root of rises in allergies. Hay fever is unknown amongst South African Xhosa tribespeople, like these women, who remain in the homelands. When they migrate to the cities, however, the children begin to show high rates of hay fever.

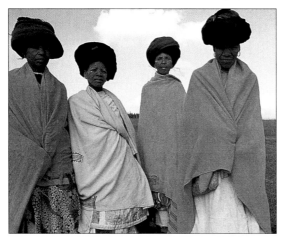

discipline of clinical ecology (known as environmental medicine in the UK), and was immediately marginalised by a suspicious medical establishment. Despite this, the environmental hypothesis (as it is known in some circles) has continued to gain strength as the incidence of all kinds of allergies has rocketed.

THE SCALE OF THE PROBLEM

While environmental allergists agree with conventional allergists on the theory of what constitutes an allergy, they disagree over how the available evidence fits into that theory (see Chapter 1). As a result, environmental allergists are far more open-minded about what can cause allergy and those conditions which may result from an allergy.

What is not in dispute by either side is that the scale of the problem is growing and that allergies now affect large numbers of the world's population. In Sweden 46 per cent of a group of 1,050 medical students were reported to have current or past allergies. In London, 46 per cent of adults tested had a positive allergy skin test in 1988, twice as many as in 1974, a doubling in only 14 years.

Figures for food allergies and chemical sensitivities are hard to come by, as few governmental health institutions recognise them as clinically authenticated conditions. But the data for what might be termed 'classical allergies' – conditions like hay fever and asthma – tell the story just as clearly.

The first case of hay fever was described in medical literature in the early 1800s and the disease has since become increasingly common. In the UK there has been a fourfold increase in rhinitis in the last 20 years, to the point where it now affects 17 per cent of the population. Clinical experience suggests that there have also been increases in many other allergy-related chronic disorders. What lies behind these extraordinary figures?

THE ENVIRONMENTAL HYPOTHESIS

Although the increase in these chronic illnesses started in the West, it is now spreading to Third World countries as they become more developed. Could elements of the modern lifestyle be responsible? Environmental allergists offer several hypotheses which relate to our diet and environment, and to how we are changing them.

Perhaps the most wide-ranging change has been the make-up of our diets. Some allergists believe that we evolved over hundreds of thousands of years to eat only what we could hunt or gather – in other words the diet consumed by our Stone Age ancestors. Since the introduction of agriculture – and more recently, modern storage methods and rapid worldwide transport – the elements of our diet have changed to include many foods that were not available in the past, or were available only rarely, and that the human body is therefore possibly ill-equipped to deal with. These include milk, eggs, potatoes and cereals, not to mention preservatives and additives. This theory could explain why these top the lists of trigger foods (see Chapter 4).

Human activities are causing the build-up of several different types of pollution, including outdoor pollution – industrial and traffic fumes; indoor pollution – from gas cookers, cigarette smoke, synthetic fabrics, pets, moulds and dust mites; food and water contamination – pesticides, fertilisers and additives; and pharmaceuticals – from drugs and medication, perfumes and make-up. As well as drastically increasing the level of potential chemical triggers to which we are exposed, there is evidence that such pollution could be changing the nature of our immune systems to make us more susceptible to allergies (see Chapter 3).

CAVEMAN CUISINE
Foods such as fresh fish and meat, certain fruits, tubers and many herbs are believed to be the sort of things our Stone Age forebears would have eaten, and thus the foods which our digestions are evolutionarily equipped to deal with.

WHAT DO DIFFERENT THERAPIES HAVE TO OFFER?

Although there are many conventional drugs and medications available for the treatment of disorders like hay fever, asthma and eczema, many patients find that these drugs provide only temporary relief, need to be taken in increasing doses (with increasingly more serious side effects) and may even cause problems themselves. In addition, most doctors do not recognise many chronic ailments as allergic, and depend on medication to suppress the symptoms without treating the underlying causes.

For many people, complementary treatments offer a gentler and more natural alternative to conventional medication, and there are many different therapies that can help with allergies. Herbal remedies can be used to treat internal disorders, as well as soothing skin

STEAM RELIEF
A face sauna clears the sinuses and helps to wash away irritating pollen. Natural remedies like this can provide alternatives to drugs in the management of rhinitis and other allergic conditions.

problems like rashes. Aromatherapy, yoga, acupuncture and relaxation techniques may help directly with symptoms, and can also play an important role in reducing stress. As helpful as all these therapies can be, however, they are limited to alleviating symptoms, without getting to the roots of the problem.

WHAT CAN YOU DO?

There is a whole range of strategies to help you cope with and manage allergies, and to reduce the risk of developing any in the first place. Learning about allergies and potential triggers will enable you to identify the threat of allergy, find out where to look for help, pin down triggers, and know how best to avoid them.

Fighting Allergies provides the information you need to help you achieve this. The emphasis of the book is on practical steps you can take, and on the therapies, both conventional and complementary, that you can use to treat and alleviate symptoms. Chapter 1 provides an explanation of the biology of allergies as well as a guide to the various methods used to test for and diagnose them. Chapter 2 gives an overview of the strategies available for treating allergies, both conventional and alternative.

The next five chapters deal with the different groups of allergen that you might encounter, and the disorders related to them. Chapter 3 covers airborne allergens, from dust mites and pollen, to chemicals and vapours, and includes the two major allergic disorders of respiration – hay fever and asthma. Chapter 4 discusses the controversial subject of food allergy, and explains how diet can cause or cure a whole range of problems. Chapter 5 looks at allergic reactions of the skin, with particular focus on the substances that we come into contact with, and the problems of eczema, dermatitis and urticaria. Chapter 6 considers drug allergies, and how to reduce need for medication so that we can avoid the attendant problems. Chapter 7 gives a round up of other sources of allergic triggers, including insects, and focuses on the deadliest of all allergic reactions – anaphylaxis.

Chapter 8 looks at the special problems of children and allergies, in particular the issue of hyperactivity and related disorders.

Finally, Chapter 9 offers a directory of allergic disorders, a ready reference guide to help you find the information you need about an illness, how allergies might be involved and how to treat and prevent allergic health problems.

T'AI CHI
The relaxing and energy boosting benefits of t'ai chi, an ancient form of oriental martial art, have been proven to help relieve a range of conditions including asthma.

Are you clued-up about allergies?

Allergy is a complicated subject about which many people, including doctors, are underinformed. For people suffering from chronic illnesses and debilitating attacks, this lack of knowledge can be very serious. Learning about allergies could be the most important step you can take to safeguard your health.

Q **DO YOU HAVE CONSTANT, UNEXPLAINED SYMPTOMS?**
If you feel ill all the time, but your symptoms are vague and ill-defined, and your doctor is at a loss, you might do well to consider the possibility of allergies. Many allergy patients are what doctors call 'thick-file' patients, because they have bulging medical files filled with notes on past ailments which did not seem to have any physical cause. Are you continually going to your GP with symptoms such as fatigue, unexplained fevers, aches and pains, mood swings, disappearing and reappearing rashes and itches and intermittent digestive upsets, but the doctor can never find much wrong with you? If so, the doctor might label you as a difficult patient, or dismiss your symptoms as psychosomatic. Chapter 2 tells you where to get help to find out if you have an allergy, and Chapter 9 explains why some doctors are reluctant to entertain the notion that allergies could be causing diverse but unrelated symptoms.

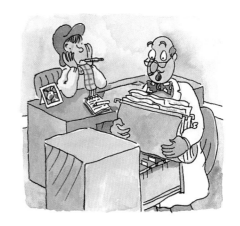

Q **SHOULD YOU BE WORRIED ABOUT ALLERGIES?**
Media interest in cases of individuals with multiple allergies (see Chapter 7) may cause concern to people who suspect they may be allergic too. Issues such as what you can safely eat may also be worrying, but before attributing your symptoms to allergy you need to look at the evidence. There are many clues which suggest allergy, but few are conclusive. The sort of vague and wide-ranging symptoms described above would strongly suggest an allergy and Chapters 3 to 7 describe possible allergic symptoms in detail. Chapter 8 outlines the markers that parents should look out for when considering whether their children have allergies. Professionals can call on a range of tests to help them diagnose allergies, from prick and patch tests to more alternative techniques like kinesiology (see Chapter 1).The best route to diagnosis is via double-blind trials of foods and chemicals, possibly following special diets which eliminate allergenic foods (see Chapters 1 and 4).

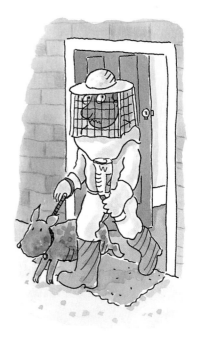

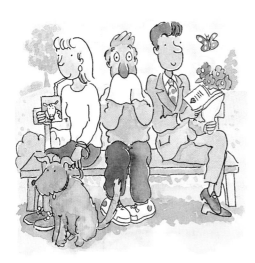

Q WHY DO ONLY SOME PEOPLE HAVE ALLERGIES?

This is a complicated issue which even the experts cannot fully answer. Genetics definitely plays some part, but exactly how, and how large a part, is not clear, especially for the more contentious types of allergy (see Chapter 1). Early exposures to potential triggers in the first years of life – including your time in the womb – are very important. This means that what your mother ate, drank and came into contact with could be vital in determining your present allergic status (see Chapters 1 and 8). Frequency of contact is also important – the most common allergens tend to be the most ubiquitous ones, a trait which applies to almost all types of allergen (see Chapters 3 to 6).

Q WHY DOESN'T MY GP BELIEVE IN FOOD ALLERGY?

All physicians recognise the existence of immediate reactions to foods, such as anaphylactic shock in reaction to eating a peanut. But delayed food reactions, where foods can cause symptoms not normally associated with the gut – such as arthritis, mood swings or fluid retention – after a gap of several hours, or even days, are a different matter. Despite a wealth of evidence to the contrary, many doctors dismiss the idea that foods can produce such reactions. Even doctors sympathetic to the idea of food allergy may only consider a limited range of potential triggers. You may need to raise the issue yourself, in which case you will need to know as much as possible about food allergy and triggers, and you may even need to know where to find alternative professional support. Chapter 4 gives detailed information on where to find help for a food allergy.

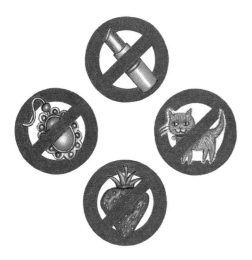

Q WHAT CAN I DO TO EASE MY SYMPTOMS?

Once you have determined which substances trigger your allergic reactions the first step should be to minimise your contact with them. In some instances this can be quite simple, for example if the allergy is to a certain make-up, you can simply stop using the make-up. Other allergies, such as those to certain foods, can be more disruptive and involve special diets and the need to shop and cook with the allergy in mind (see Chapter 4). Perhaps the most difficult allergies to cope with are those to the environment, such as reactions to pollens, or chemicals in the air. Avoiding pollen, dust mites, chemicals and pet dander is difficult, but even here there are precautions you can take and treatments that will help provide relief from symptoms (see Chapter 3).

CHAPTER 1

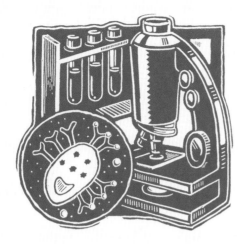

EXPLAINING ALLERGIES

Ever since allergies were first recognised in the early part of the century they have attracted controversy. What constitutes an allergy, which substances can cause one, and how should a sufferer be treated? This chapter attempts to present the basic knowledge that you will need to understand who means what by the term 'allergy'.

WHAT IS AN ALLERGY?

Even the definition of the word allergy is fraught with controversy. Health practitioners from different professional backgrounds mean different things when they use the term.

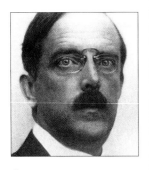

CLEMENS VON PIRQUET (1874–1924)
This Austrian physician coined the term 'allergy' in 1906. He used it to describe an abnormal reaction by the body to a normally harmless foreign substance.

THE UNLIKELY ENEMY
In an allergic reaction normally harmless substances, such as dried cat saliva, can produce damaging immune responses.

Many people have experienced an allergic reaction: developing a rash after using a new suntan cream or sneezing on entering a dusty room and most hay fever sufferers understand that their symptoms are brought on in the summer months by pollen. There may also be more subtle kinds of allergic reaction where symptoms are delayed or hidden. Some allergies to foods are examples of this.

But why should an apparently harmless substance such as a pollen grain cause such a severe reaction?

ALLERGY AND THE IMMUNE SYSTEM

Doctors have learnt that in reactions such as hay fever or eczema it is the body's immune system that causes the symptoms. What seems to happen in an allergic reaction is that a substance, such as pollen, which should present no threat to the body, is seen as hostile by the immune system. The 'invader' is expelled, by sneezing, coughing, a runny nose or weeping rash.

To properly understand what an allergy is, a basic understanding of the immune system – its components, and how they work together – is essential. The role of the immune system is to protect us from potentially harmful substances and organisms that could cause disease or infection. It is composed of several different types of cells and molecules which are present in blood and tissues, especially in parts of the body that are exposed to the external environment, for example the eyes. These cells and molecules are able to recognise hostile organisms or foreign material and retaliate by producing defensive weapons directed specifically at the invader.

Antibodies and immune cells

Antibodies are the 'foot-soldiers' of the immune system. They serve to recognise and identify foreign organisms and substances, attack them directly and interact with other cells in the immune system to destroy invaders. A new-born baby is equipped with some antibodies from its mother, but most are produced after birth.

Antibodies are found in the blood and other body fluids. They are proteins whose structure is precisely engineered to fit the surface components of germs, like a key fits into a lock. Antibodies are more precisely termed immunoglobulins (abbreviated to Ig) and are divided into sub-classes which are termed IgA, IgD, IgE, IgG and IgM.

Each class of antibody works in a somewhat different way and has a different job to do. Some cause the release of large numbers of chemical messengers, others bind to the target germs and cause them to clump together to make larger clumps which then attract white blood cells such as phagocytes.

IgE antibodies are particularly important in allergic reactions. They coat mast cells and basophils (types of immune cell), acting as receptors – molecules on the surface of a cell that recognise and bind to passing molecules, and trigger changes inside the cell.

When an invading allergen (any substance, particle or organism that provokes an allergic response) binds to these IgE receptors, the mast cells or basophils are triggered to release their cargo of inflammatory messenger chemicals, such as histamine, producing inflammation.

ELEMENTS OF THE IMMUNE SYSTEM

The immune system is composed of cells and molecules whose function is to identify, attack and destroy invaders. However, each of these elements can be triggered by harmless substances as well as germs. When this happens, and allergic symptoms result, it is called allergy as opposed to immunity.

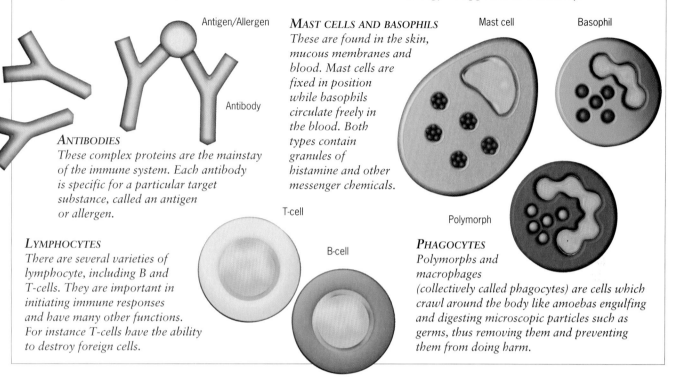

ANTIBODIES
These complex proteins are the mainstay of the immune system. Each antibody is specific for a particular target substance, called an antigen or allergen.

MAST CELLS AND BASOPHILS
These are found in the skin, mucous membranes and blood. Mast cells are fixed in position while basophils circulate freely in the blood. Both types contain granules of histamine and other messenger chemicals.

LYMPHOCYTES
There are several varieties of lymphocyte, including B and T-cells. They are important in initiating immune responses and have many other functions. For instance T-cells have the ability to destroy foreign cells.

PHAGOCYTES
Polymorphs and macrophages (collectively called phagocytes) are cells which crawl around the body like amoebas engulfing and digesting microscopic particles such as germs, thus removing them and preventing them from doing harm.

Inflammation brings immune cells into the area, provides the optimal temperature for their activity and flushes the affected tissue with fluid to help wash away germs or allergens and the debris of cell damage.

Other important cells in the immune system include phagocytes which engulf and digest smaller particles and germs, and lymphocytes. Lymphocytes are the heavy artillery of the immune system, that may be called upon in particularly resistant infections. They can initiate immune responses and attack foreign cells directly. Some types of lymphocyte, known as B-cells, can turn into antibody factories, secreting the various types of immunoglobin into the blood.

Complement is the name given to a group of normal blood proteins which can be activated during an immune reaction. Part of their function is to kill bacteria and other cells after they have been coated by antibodies. Once activated by antibodies, they also serve to induce inflammation.

Although this is by no means the complete cast list of the immune system, it covers the elements essential to the production of an allergic reaction.

THE PHYSIOLOGY OF AN ALLERGY

The different forces of the immune system outlined above are marshalled into several lines of defence. Where tissues are in direct contact with the outside world – the skin,

THE LYMPHATIC SYSTEM

The lymphatic system is an important part of the body's immune system. It consists of a set of vessels which collect lymph fluid from the tissues of the body and drain it back into the blood. Lymph nodes are situated throughout the lymphatic system, and act as a barrier to the spread of infection, destroying or filtering out bacteria and other harmful agents.

LYMPH FLUID
Lymph is a clear fluid composed of water, protein and sundry other substances, but most importantly it carries white blood cells.

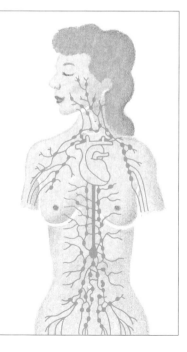

During a Type I allergic reaction, mast cells are triggered into degranulating. Chemicals like histamine, normally stored as granules within the cell, are released, causing inflammation and attracting other immune cells.

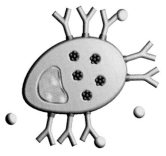

Step 1 IgE antibodies adhere to receptors on the membrane of the mast cell. Each is specific for an allergen.

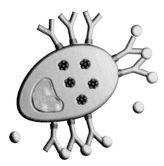

Step 2 The antibodies react with allergens, activating the mast cell.

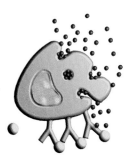

Step 3 The mast cell degranulates releasing its cargo of inflammatory chemicals.

the respiratory and intestinal tracts, and so on – various elements of the immune system are concentrated. For instance, mast cells and basophils will be anchored in the connective tissues of the skin and the lining of the lungs, phagocytes will patrol in the blood, the mucus of the sinuses and the tear ducts of the eyes, and antibodies can be found almost everywhere in the body.

If an allergen is seen as a risk by the immune system – for example when a bee sting injects venom into the skin, or pollen gets into the mucus of the lungs – one or other of the elements of the immune system recognises the invading substance, or some part of it, as a hostile entity. This sets in motion a train of events that may include the release of chemical messengers such as histamine or heparin, the activation of complement or the attack of killer T-cells. This will not happen on the first exposure to an allergen, because the immune system needs at least one exposure to become sensitised to a specific allergen.

Immunologists recognise four types of immune response to allergens. Each is defined in terms of the mechanism involved, rather than the symptoms produced.

Type I allergy

This is caused mostly by antibodies of the IgE class which are found on the surface of cells such as basophils and mast cells. When this antibody recognises the precise antigen that it was made for, and binds to it, it causes histamine and other inflammatory substances to be released from the cells. The result is inflammation in which reddening and itchiness are major features.

IgE antibodies appear to have few beneficial effects, except perhaps for helping to rid the body of worms and other parasites, which are not a major problem in the developed world. When Type I allergy affects the moist membranes of the eyes, nose, lungs or intestine another feature is the production of mucus (runny nose, phlegm) and involuntary expulsive efforts (sneezing, coughing, vomiting or scratching, depending on which organ is affected). This type of allergy matches most closely with what environmental allergists term Type A allergy (see page 20).

Type I allergy is also known as 'atopy'. An individual is said to be atopic when he or she overproduces IgE. This means that IgE is at a raised level in the blood and on

INFLAMMATION

This is the body's natural response to invaders or foreign substances which have not been fully dealt with by the immune system, and have started to cause damage. Inflammation is recognised by its five cardinal signs: swelling of the area, redness, heat, pain and impaired function. Histamine and other chemical messengers cause the capillaries – the tiny blood vessels in the skin – to dilate, stretching their walls so that fluid and immune cells leak into the surrounding tissues and deal with invaders.

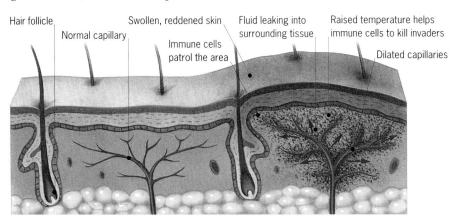

Skin without inflammation – normal colour and temperature. There are no unusual raised areas or swelling or unusual immune activity.

Inflamed skin – reddened, warmed surface of the skin. Leaky capillaries cause swelling as fluid builds up. Immune cells patrol the area.

mast cells, so that the sufferer is always reactive to even low levels of whatever allergen stimulated the antibody production in the first place – for instance mould spores, chemicals, pollen or house dust which are all present in the atmosphere.

As a result the sufferers have an allergic reaction, such as asthma, eczema, urticaria or rhinitis, whenever they are exposed to the allergen, which may be a seasonal occurrence, or may happen constantly. A classic example would be hay fever, in which allergy to airborne pollen grains causes the eyes and nose to become inflamed (conjunctivitis and rhinitis).

Type II allergy

This is caused by antibodies of the IgG or IgM class when they combine with complement to kill antigenic cells (cells that the immune system sees as invaders). One example is drug-induced anaemia. This is where a particular drug binds to the surface of the patient's red blood cells and causes them to become antigenic, so that the immune system regards them as foreign. This leads to the production of antibodies, which are called 'autoantibodies' because they are directed against the body's own cells rather than foreign cells. These antibodies are actually directed against the drug molecules stuck to the cells' surfaces, but the effect nonetheless is to activate complement, which causes the red blood cells to break up, resulting in anaemia. This type of allergy is rare.

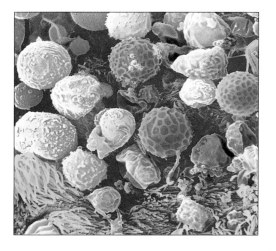

Type III allergy

This is again caused by IgG or IgM antibodies and complement. The damage is caused by the inflammatory action of complement. The type of inflammation is slower than Type I inflammation, and lasts longer. The area does not itch much but is very tender. The classic example of a Type III reaction would be farmer's lung, caused by the inhalation of fungal spores during the handling of damp hay, which causes inflammation of the lungs. Occupational exposure to mould spores also causes cheese washer's disease, furrier's lung and maple bark stripper's lung.

Type IV allergy

This is not caused by antibodies but by lymphocytes of the kind known as 'killer cells'. These cells can kill invading microorganisms externally, without having to

RESPIRATORY INVADERS
Minute particles like the pollen, dust and mould spores shown here can build up in the lungs of people whose jobs expose them to substances like damp, mouldy hay or flour. After prolonged exposure, Type III allergic reactions can cause conditions like farmer's lung.

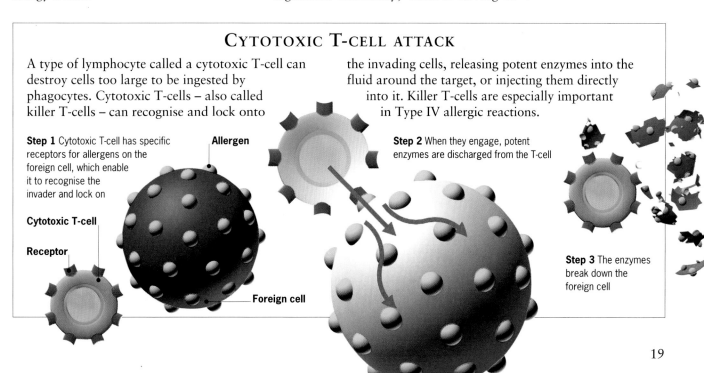

CYTOTOXIC T-CELL ATTACK

A type of lymphocyte called a cytotoxic T-cell can destroy cells too large to be ingested by phagocytes. Cytotoxic T-cells – also called killer T-cells – can recognise and lock onto the invading cells, releasing potent enzymes into the fluid around the target, or injecting them directly into it. Killer T-cells are especially important in Type IV allergic reactions.

Step 1 Cytotoxic T-cell has specific receptors for allergens on the foreign cell, which enable it to recognise the invader and lock on

Allergen

Cytotoxic T-cell

Receptor

Step 2 When they engage, potent enzymes are discharged from the T-cell

Step 3 The enzymes break down the foreign cell

Foreign cell

Taking sides
In the UK, conventional allergists are represented by the British Society for Allergy and Clinical Immunology, while environmental allergists are represented by the British Society for Allergy, Environmental and Nutritional Medicine. Some allergists are members of both.

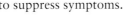

A DIFFERENCE OF APPROACH

Conventional allergists look specifically at whether the patient has IgE antibodies to allergens, and mostly use medication to suppress symptoms.

Environmental allergists consider a wider range of symptom triggers and mainly advise on avoidance and protection to prevent the symptoms.

CONVENTIONAL
The history of the patient's symptoms (for example rhinitis) leads to blood tests and skin prick tests to confirm allergy – but usually only Type I allergy, involving IgE. Drugs may then be prescribed to suppress the symptoms.

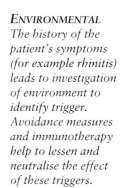

ENVIRONMENTAL
The history of the patient's symptoms (for example rhinitis) leads to investigation of environment to identify trigger. Avoidance measures and immunotherapy help to lessen and neutralise the effect of these triggers.

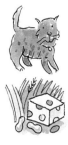

ingest them first. A Type IV reaction can result in scarring, if severe enough. A classic example of a mild Type IV allergy is contact allergy to the nickel in some jewellery. Type IV responses can also cause other types of hypersensitive reactions involving diseases like tuberculosis and leprosy.

DIFFERENT SCHOOLS OF THOUGHT

Allergists fall into two schools of thought: conventional allergists and environmental allergists (also known as clinical ecologists). They differ primarily over the issue of what constitutes an allergic reaction, and what does not. But this central dispute also leads to disagreements on questions such as which substances can act as allergens, and which health conditions are allergic.

The conventional approach

Conventional and environmental allergists agree that reactions that do not have an immunological mechanism are not allergies. But conventional allergists go further: they hold that any condition that has not been clearly shown to conform to one of the four types of mechanism is not an allergy. In practice it is not unusual for patients who are found to be negative for Type I allergy to be told that their problems are not allergic. Even in the most strict scientific terms this may not be true because a lot of work is still needed to establish – or rule out – the involvement of the Types II, III and IV

mechanisms and most of the tests that conventional allergists consider reliable enough to use only apply to Type I allergies.

The environmental approach

Environmental allergists start by establishing that environmental influences make the patient ill and that avoiding exposure makes a substantial difference to their well-being. This occurs in two patterns which they refer to as Type A and intolerance. However, because many of the cases referred to as intolerance have features suggestive of immunological mechanisms, environmental allergists give them the benefit of the doubt and call them Type B allergies.

TYPE A AND TYPE B ALLERGIES

Generally speaking, Type A allergies include most of the types recognised by immunologists, for instance hay fever. Type B allergies show some characteristics of immune reactions, for instance they are specific to particular allergens, and they may eventually be shown to be due to Type III or IV mechanisms. But unlike Type A symptoms they often have delayed effects, or effects in other parts of the body.

For example, inhaling some pollen could lead to gut pains, aching joints or eczema, none of which are symptoms typically associated with pollen allergy. Equally an allergy to a food might cause symptoms in a part of the body not associated with the mouth or gut – nasal symptoms, like rhinitis, for

PSEUDOALLERGIES

Pseudoallergy is the clinical term for a reaction where the trigger has a direct effect on the mast cells and basophils. This direct effect causes the cells to degranulate (see page 18) and release histamine and other inflammatory substances. In other words antibodies and other parts of the immune system are not involved, which means that the reaction is not allergic. However, the effects are the same, and avoiding the trigger prevents the symptoms, just as with an allergy, so it is not always clear whether a substance is having a direct pseudoallergic effect, or an immune-mediated allergic effect.

instance. The symptoms might take several hours to develop and if the food is eaten often it will never be clear that there is a link between eating the food and the onset of nasal symptoms. Both of these examples would be Type B reactions.

Intolerance

Other types of reaction are intolerances due to a shortage of enzymes or to chronic toxicity. These are not allergies. Since it is not always easy to differentiate, however, some people refer to Type B reactions as intolerances. Conventional allergists argue that intolerance and other non-allergic mechanisms underlie most Type B reactions. Environmental allergists disagree, and this is the source of some of the most bitter controversy in the field.

Other types of reaction

Symptoms that closely resemble Type A or Type B symptoms can also be produced by other non-allergic reactions such as chronic toxicity or pseudoallergy. Alternative practitioners sometimes use the term allergy more loosely to include such reactions, and, in fact, conditions in real life are rarely clear cut, often containing elements of several different phenomena.

Strengths and weaknesses

The differences between conventional and environmental allergists arise, in part, because the former base their classification on underlying mechanisms rather than symptoms, while the latter use symptoms and their response to treatment, not mechanisms, as a guide. Also, immunologists and conventional allergists rely on laboratory findings for diagnosis, while there are no easy laboratory tests for a Type B allergy. The range of the symptoms differs too.

Both systems of classification have their strengths and weaknesses, and the wise allergist needs to have both in mind. Unfortunately, there is still disagreement. Conventional allergists are well trained in immunology but tend not to notice intolerances. If they fail to find evidence of immune system involvement they are in danger of dismissing a very real illness.

Doctors of the environmental medicine (or clinical ecology) school, on the other hand, tend not to be concerned with the biological mechanisms involved and are more interested in what happens to patients when suspect items are eliminated and then reintroduced, whether this is done in the clinic or at home, by the patients themselves.

Masked allergy

In particular, the environmental medicine approach recognises a condition called 'masked allergy' which conventional allergists do not acknowledge. Some practitioners argue that some forms of masked allergy are actually a type of food addiction. See Chapter 4 for more details.

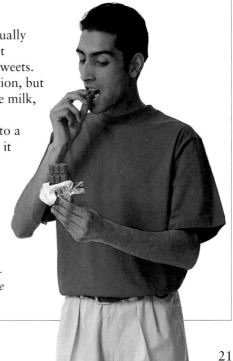

FOOD ADDICTION

Addictions to food are actually quite common, and are not restricted to caffeine and sweets. Any food can cause addiction, but the commonest culprits are milk, wheat, cheese, nuts and chocolate. Being addicted to a food means that removing it from the diet can provoke withdrawal symptoms.

PRIME SUSPECTS
Foods which elicit strong feelings – and this includes both cravings and aversions – should be considered as prime food allergy suspects.

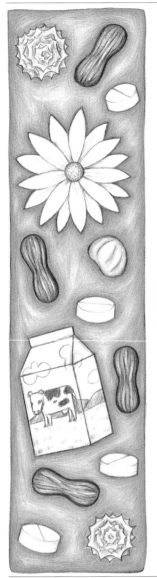

CONTROVERSY IN THE WORLD OF ALLERGIES

Immunologists (including conventional allergists) and environmental allergists disagree over several issues, and use the term allergy differently. Immunologists use allergy to mean an immune-mediated reaction, while environmental allergists use it to mean the harmful effect of an environmental or dietary substance, which has features indicating or proving that it is caused by an immunological reaction. The latter group classify allergies on the basis of clinical pattern, while the former use the four types of immunological reaction. Immunologists restrict the list of conditions that they consider allergic to reactions such as hay fever, asthma and eczema. Environmental allergists include all these, together with arthritis, migraine, weight fluctuation, hyperactivity, irritable bowel syndrome and many others. Immunologists test for allergies using defined tests, but environmental allergists have no reliable laboratory diagnostic method. Both groups advocate the avoidance of allergens; immunologists also use drug treatment while environmental allergists avoid drugs where possible (see Chapter 2).

CONTROVERSIAL AREA	IMMUNOLOGISTS	ENVIRONMENTAL ALLERGISTS
Meaning of 'allergy'	Immune-mediated reaction (i.e. caused by the action of the immune system)	Sensitivity to an environmental or dietary substance with features which suggest allergy
Classification of allergies	Types I-V immunology	Types A and B based on pattern of symptoms and response to avoidance
What conditions might be allergic	Hay fever, asthma, eczema, urticaria, anaphylaxis	All these plus arthritis, migraine, mood disorders and many others
Methods of diagnosis	Tests of immune function	Avoidance and challenge (see page 33). No reliable laboratory diagnostic tests – diagnosis based on history or made in retrospect
Methods of treatment (see Chapter 2)	Avoidance of allergen or drug treatment, desensitisation (for venom allergies) (see Chapter 2)	Avoidance of allergen or desensitisation to a range of allergens

ALLERGIC SYMPTOMS

The most familiar allergic symptoms are those that environmental allergists would classify as Type A – they tend to be short, sharp and discrete in onset and effect. Type B symptoms are more likely to be chronic and vague, and often appear to be unconnected with the trigger or triggers.

Type A symptoms

Most people are familiar with the classic symptoms of well-known allergies such as hay fever or peanut allergy. The systems affected by these are the body's most vulnerable: the skin and the respiratory and gastrointestinal systems.

Sneezing, coughing and excessive production of mucus causing a runny nose and phlegm are obvious characteristics of Type A allergies. A more severe problem is asthma, where the airways constrict and become filled with mucus, making breathing difficult (see page 72). Asthma ranges in severity and is rarely fatal, but it is becoming more common, particularly among children and young adults. Some children grow out of it. Eye problems – allergic conjunctivitis – including itching, swelling and watering are common Type A symptoms, especially with allergy to animals.

Foods and antibiotics often cause gastrointestinal problems, such as vomiting, diarrhoea or abdominal pain. In Type A conditions these symptoms come on almost immediately. They may also be accompanied by skin problems – eczema and urticaria. The immediacy of effect makes it relatively easy to identify the trigger.

Eczema, or dermatitis, may be a Type A reaction. Initially there is an increased blood flow to the affected area, causing redness. This is followed by itchiness and the formation of blisters, which may rupture and cause weeping. The skin becomes thickened and flaky, and this may be chronic.

Urticaria, also called nettle-rash or hives, involves swelling and discoloration of the skin. The swelling can be either deep-seated or superficial. The latter is common in Type A allergies, and although usually acute and short-lived, it can be very irritating. Deeper swelling, known as angio-oedema, is often associated with allergenic foods, and is mostly restricted to the face, lips, tongue and throat. Angio-oedema comes on very quickly, sometimes immediately.

Anaphylaxis

This is a rare but potentially life-threatening condition that results from extreme sensitivity to an allergen. The most common causes are nuts, seafood, wasp and bee stings and prescription drugs like penicillin and other antibiotics. In a strictly clinical sense, anaphylaxis refers to any sort of hypersensitive reaction, and can be local and relatively mild. However, it is usually used to mean anaphylactic shock, which is a system-wide reaction. The effects are very rapid, with itching and all-over swelling leading to wheezing, collapse and possibly even heart failure. A few cases every year are fatal, but normally anaphylactic shock is not this severe and responds well to prompt treatment. Anaphylaxis usually involves IgE antibodies, in a Type I reaction, but there are alternative routes, such as the activation of complement, or non-immune pathways that mimic anaphylaxis – these are called anaphylactoid reactions, and respond to the same sort of treatment (see Chapter 7).

Chronic symptoms

Many conventional doctors and immunologists dismiss the claims made by environmental allergists that Type B allergies can cause a wide range of chronic disorders and symptoms. This dismissal is easier to understand when the number of disorders is considered. Many of the symptoms are vague and hard to pin down, such as sleeplessness or excessive sweating. Nonetheless they pose a very real problem for sufferers, who often do not get taken seriously by doctors. They may be misdiagnosed or simply dismissed as hypochondriac. Doctors even have a name for what they see as a basically psychological condition – somatisation disorder. Fortunately these symptoms usually respond well to environmental treatment – namely avoidance of the trigger – and sometimes the exact cause (that is, the allergen) does not need to be identified for treatment to be effective (see Chapter 2).

Symptoms of Type B conditions
Type B conditions can involve a wide range of disorders, affecting almost every system in the body. These include: fatigue and lethargy; heartburn; sleeplessness; catarrh and sinus problems; cold hands and feet; constant runny nose; diarrhoea or constipation (or both); sore lips, gums, eyes, tongue; wind; weight fluctuation, bloating, obesity; chronic indigestion; skin and hair problems; migraine and other headaches; muscle, joint and bone ache; arthritis; excessive sweating; hyperactivity; cystitis; depression and irritability; stress incontinence; asthma; and period problems.

SYMPTOMS OF TYPES A AND B REACTIONS

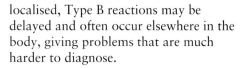

The key differences between the symptoms of Type A and Type B allergic reactions are that while most Type A symptoms occur immediately and are localised, Type B reactions may be delayed and often occur elsewhere in the body, giving problems that are much harder to diagnose.

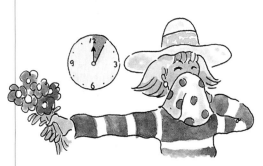

IMMEDIATE
Type A symptoms tend to appear at or near the point of contact with an allergen – for example swollen eyes or sneezing.

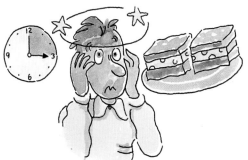

DELAYED
Type B symptoms, such as migraine, may appear soon after contact with an allergen, but often take hours or days to come on.

COMMON ALLERGENS

The substance that causes an allergic reaction is termed the allergen. There are thousands of known allergens, of which a few dozen are particularly notorious troublemakers.

Virtually any substance can cause allergy, but there is a 'league table', with very common problem substances at one end and very rare allergy triggers at the other.

WHAT MAKES A SUBSTANCE ALLERGENIC?

To a large extent the frequency with which a substance causes allergy depends on how much of it there is in our lives. Cow's milk heads the list of foods causing Type B allergies, probably because it is encountered so early in life, and in the Western world is widely consumed by adults, mostly every day. But milk allergy is extremely rare in China, where hardly any adults consume it because of their genetic inability to digest lactose, the sugar found in milk.

The people factor

The way in which allergy has emerged as a problem over the past 200 years suggests that another factor – something in the modern environment – is important in determining how individuals respond to allergens.

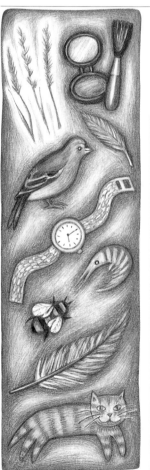

COMMON ALLERGENS

Allergens can be categorised by their route of contact and by their biological or chemical nature. In the table below the most common allergens are divided into the most useful groupings frequently used in diagnosis and treatment. As the table shows, allergens that cause Type A reactions can also cause Type B ones.

NATURE OF ALLERGEN	ROUTE OF CONTACT	ALLERGENS CAUSING TYPE A AND B REACTIONS	ALLERGENS CAUSING TYPE B REACTIONS
Aeroallergens	Inhaled	Grass pollens, tree and plant pollens, dust mite allergens, mould spores, wool fibres, feathers, some chemicals	Inhaled chemical pollutants and volatile organic chemicals (VOCs)
Food	Ingested or contact	Mainly shellfish, fish, eggs, nuts, peanuts	All foods, especially those eaten frequently – milk, wheat, other grains, citrus fruits Food additives such as colourings, flavourings and preservatives Food contaminants
Animal	Inhaled or contact	Dogs, cats, horses, rabbits, guinea pigs, birds	
Biting/ stinging insects	Bites or stings	Wasps, bees, mosquitoes, hornets, horseflies	
Drugs	Ingested, injected or applied	Various, e.g. antibiotics	Many drugs and their fillers, colourings and preservatives
Other	On contact	Latex, nickel and other metals, semen, make-up	

Since the Industrial Revolution there has been a vast increase in the levels of synthesised and polluting chemicals that we breathe, eat and drink. Industrial countries have noticed marked increases in both Type A and Type B allergy symptoms in the past 50 years, and levels are rising in less developed countries as they become industrialised. It certainly seems as if there is a link between environmental change and allergies in general (see Chapter 3 for more details). However, such a link does not explain which substances cause problems and why.

The raw and the cooked

There are several factors that help to determine whether a food causes problems. In particular some foods change their allergenic properties depending on how they are prepared.

Cooking can change the reactive properties of some foods – for instance kidney beans must be boiled hard to get rid of toxins, and some allergens in milk are broken down on heating. Milk is also altered during cheese, yoghurt or butter processing, and some people who cannot drink milk can tolerate these foods. Curing meats may involve the addition of chemicals, and processed or manufactured foods nearly always contain a host of colourings, flavourings and preservatives (see Chapter 4).

Allergens as toxins

Sometimes an allergen may have toxic effects as well as antigenic (immune reaction-causing) ones. Even pollen grains and dust mites, the classic 'harmless' allergens, are capable of bursting open and killing red blood cells, if placed close to them, and the toxins responsible are inflammatory to human skin. Clearly toxicology is important as well as immunology, although this is a controversial area where little is known.

Understanding allergic symptoms

How can we start to make sense of the apparently senseless inflammation, the 'immunity gone wrong', that constitutes Type I allergy? Sneezing, coughing, vomiting and diarrhoea are all obvious excretion mechanisms, as is the outpouring of mucus that accompanies them. Eczema and urticaria, the itchy complaints, might also enhance excretion from the skin, since the scratching that ensues should encourage

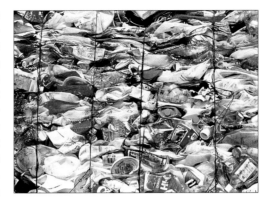

lymph flow and perhaps excretion of trigger substances through the skin itself in the weeping fluid of eczema. Asthma, which restricts air intake into the lungs, will prevent entry of allergenic particles and germs and encourage turbulent air flow in breathing out, which in turn increases the passage of mucus out of the lungs.

Type A allergic symptoms, in this view, represent the body's attempts (usually successful) to expel potentially harmful particles and gases from the body. Type B symptoms could be taken as a sign that these attempts are ineffective, that the body's defence systems have been overwhelmed or were not strong enough in the first place. This raises questions such as 'why?' and 'what can be done about it?', particularly as the incidence of Type B allergic conditions is rising so fast. These questions cannot be properly answered at present, but improved nutrition and lessened exposure to chemicals might help to slow this rise, particularly in the very young.

None of this means that doctors should not try to treat and alleviate allergic symptoms. But it should dictate a note of caution in therapy: itching and wheezing may be doing a useful job, so rather than exerting efforts to suppress symptoms, try to find out the underlying causes of their provocation.

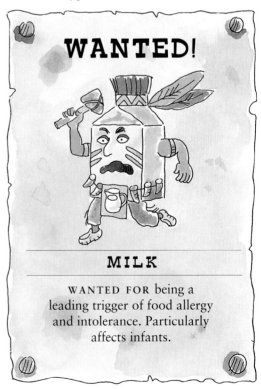

WANTED!

MILK

WANTED FOR being a leading trigger of food allergy and intolerance. Particularly affects infants.

WHO GETS ALLERGIES AND WHY?

Although genetics plays a part in allergy susceptibility, it can be hard to separate its role from that played by environmental factors, particularly around the time of birth.

ARE ALLERGIES HEREDITARY?

Type I allergies (the most well understood ones) tend to run in families, though the genetics are complex and have not yet been exactly worked out.

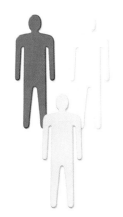

A person with one atopic parent (see Glossary) has perhaps a 35 per cent chance of developing Type I allergies.

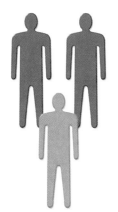

If both parents are atopic the probability rises to around 70 per cent.

Biological characteristics are determined by a combination of genetic and environmental factors, and allergies are no exception. The months before and after birth are a vulnerable period during which babies can develop allergies. But this is an area under investigated by scientists, and while much is known, much remains obscure. It is known that having an immune system which is sensitive to normally harmless substances is partly a matter of heredity (see below), particularly with Type I allergy, or atopy. Equally, many studies show that there is a window of vulnerability during the months before and after birth, when a susceptible individual can become sensitised to allergens. Sensitisation can happen throughout life, but becomes less likely with age. Thus environmental factors interact with a genetic predisposition to determine the final extent and severity of an individual's allergies.

HOW COMMON ARE ALLERGIC CONDITIONS?

Estimates vary depending on which conditions are considered to be allergic, but the most conservative estimate is that they affect about 10-20 per cent of the population (mainly asthma, eczema and hay fever). If the conditions classed as Type B are included, this estimate would more than double. American allergist William Rea suggests, plausibly, that the allergy patients who come to doctors represent the tip of a very large iceberg, and that mild degrees of allergic illness are so common that only very few people are completely well and functioning at full potential. Certainly experienced allergists see mild cases all around them, among family and friends – as the famous English physician Richard Asher put it, 'allergists see the world through allergy-coloured spectacles'. It seems probable that most people's health could be improved by careful attention to diet and environment.

Twins

In pairs of identical twins, one may have a severe Type I allergic illness and the other not, even though the unaffected twin has positive IgE and skin tests, so obviously there are other factors at work. Once an individual has the genetic potential to become allergic, several environmental trigger factors may be needed to cause the development of allergy.

Infant exposure

The first few weeks of life are crucial. If babies are kept away from dust, furry animals and allergenic foods during this time, they are less likely to develop Type I aller-

NATURE OR NURTURE?

Children inherit far more than genes from their parents; they also inherit dietary and lifestyle habits. This makes it hard for scientists studying the genetics of allergy to tease out the extent to which susceptibility to allergies is determined by genes, and the extent to which it depends on a person's environment, particularly their early environment. For instance, conditions in the womb are vital in determining allergies, but these conditions depend to some extent on the mother's genes.

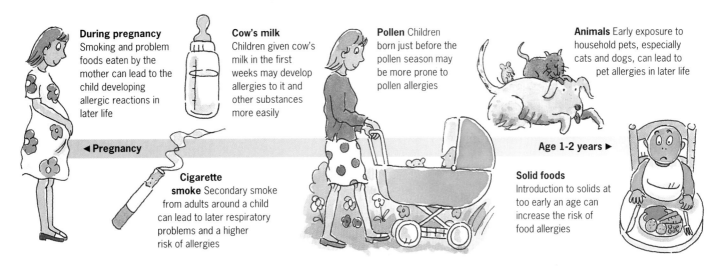

During pregnancy Smoking and problem foods eaten by the mother can lead to the child developing allergic reactions in later life

Cow's milk Children given cow's milk in the first weeks may develop allergies to it and other substances more easily

Pollen Children born just before the pollen season may be more prone to pollen allergies

Animals Early exposure to household pets, especially cats and dogs, can lead to pet allergies in later life

◄ **Pregnancy**

Age 1-2 years ►

Cigarette smoke Secondary smoke from adults around a child can lead to later respiratory problems and a higher risk of allergies

Solid foods Introduction to solids at too early an age can increase the risk of food allergies

gies in later years. The mother should avoid the same things for the last few months of pregnancy. For the first few months the baby should be fed nothing at all other than mother's milk. Babies fed other foods as well develop as many allergies as bottle-fed babies, if not more.

Tobacco smoke

This is the number one allergy trigger, especially in infancy. Tobacco smoke tends to divert the immune system into IgE production, so dusts, pollens and foods that the baby encounters during the first months are more likely to cause trouble later if he or she is exposed to smoke at the same time.

Cow's milk

There is some evidence that cow's milk can make a child more likely to become allergic to other allergens. Allergists tend to be suspicious of milk, in spite of its nutritional value, because it so often acts as an allergen itself, causing numerous childhood health problems. However milk and milk products are an excellent source of calcium and children should not be taken off milk unless their nutrition is carefully balanced.

Season of birth

Studies show that babies born in the spring months at the start of the pollen season are more likely to become allergic to pollens than those born in winter months. Again, this is because of the 'window of vulnerability' during the first weeks.

Infections and traumas

Symptoms of both Type A and Type B allergies often occur for the first time after a bout of flu or glandular fever. Type B conditions frequently follow other traumas (physical, chemical or emotional), especially when these occur closely together.

Nutrition

Modern fast food of the 'hamburgers and cola' variety, although rich in calories and proteins, tends to be poor in important vitamins and trace minerals. Although many people survive this kind of diet without apparent ill effects, they are more vulnerable to the various triggers listed above, especially if genetically predisposed to allergy. There is evidence that allergic patients are often short of trace nutrients, such as magnesium, but it is unclear whether this is a cause or a result of allergy.

HERITABILITY OF INTOLERANCES

Symptoms similar to those caused by Type B allergies may be caused by intolerances or pseudoallergies. Intolerances, such as lactose intolerance, can be caused by an enzyme deficiency (see page 78). Such a deficiency could be due in turn to a hereditary genetic factor.

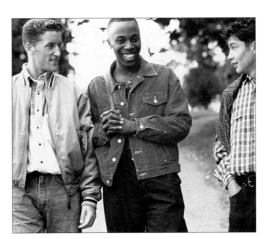

CHILDHOOD DANGERS
Expectant and breast-feeding mothers with allergies themselves (whose babies have a greater chance of being susceptible) should try to avoid foods and inhalants that they are sensitive to. All mothers should be aware of the dangers of introducing babies to allergens in the months before and after birth.

LACTOSE INTOLERANCE
Most people of Oriental or African descent are lactose intolerant (see page 78) because they are genetically programmed to stop producing lactase, the enzyme that breaks down lactose, after infancy.

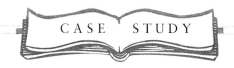
New-found Allergy Sufferer

Many allergies develop during early childhood, fade during adolescence and adulthood, but then reappear in middle and old age. Other allergies are simply not discovered until an individual has more contact with the allergen. Nickel, for instance, despite being one of the most common causes of contact allergy, may not cause trouble until relatively late in life.

On her 16th birthday Emily had her ears pierced and was given a pair of gold-coloured earrings by a friend at school. Within a few days she found that her ear lobes became itchy and inflamed. Bathing the wounds in antiseptic at home did not help, so she went to the family doctor. He diagnosed an infection, told her to stop wearing the earrings and prescribed a course of antibiotics, but the drugs did not help much and the problem with her ears did not clear up. Over the next few weeks she started to get patches of itchy, dry skin, similar to that on her ear lobes, developing elsewhere on her body – on the insides of her elbows and knees, and particularly on her wrists, and the middle of her back.

WHAT SHOULD EMILY DO?

When Emily visited her doctor again he realised that his first diagnosis had probably been wrong, and decided to refer her to an allergy specialist (see page 34). The specialist carried out a skin test to confirm his suspicions that Emily had an allergic reaction to nickel, a common component of earrings and piercing needles. The specialist advised Emily to avoid all contact with nickel in order to give her condition a chance to clear up. She needs to change her earrings and her watch strap, bracelets and bra clasp, which contain nickel and have also caused a reaction, and she must be careful from now on when handling change and choosing jewellery and clothes.

HEALTH
Allergic reactions caused by contact with an allergen can cause eczema, where the skin is flaky, itchy and develops a rash.

CLOTHING
Earrings and other jewellery frequently contain nickel, and it is found in some silver, gold (yellow and white) and platinum. It is also found in metal haberdashery like buttons and clasps.

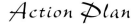

Action Plan

HEALTH
Avoiding nickel should clear up the allergic reaction.

CLOTHING
Become more conscious about day-to-day elements of lifestyle, such as the type of buttons on clothing or even handling change with sweaty hands.

LIFESTYLE
To avoid becoming sensitised to nickel in the first place, insist that ear piercing is done with a nickel-free steel needle, and then wear only pure silver or pure 18-carat gold jewellery afterwards.

HOW THINGS TURNED OUT FOR EMILY

The allergist told her that she had allergic contact eczema rather than an infection, and advised her on how to avoid nickel completely, for instance, by wearing pure silver, gold or nickel-free steel earrings. She bought a new leather watch strap and bras with plastic fastenings and got rid of some cheap jewellery she had bought as a child. Within a few weeks of taking the allergist's advice, Emily's eczema cleared up and her skin returned to normal.

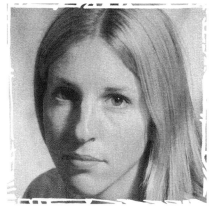

LIFESTYLE
Nickel is a very common cause of contact allergy for women, mainly due to ear piercing.

ALLERGY AND OTHER ILLNESSES

Allergic reactions have complicated short and long-term effects on many systems of the body. Naturally such effects interact with and are affected by other diseases and disorders.

Conventional medicine maintains what many allergy specialists consider to be an artificial divide between allergies and 'real illnesses'. The list of Type B symptoms includes a wide range of disorders normally considered to be 'non-allergic', but they respond to 'allergic treatment' and seem to be similar to allergies in many other significant ways. To confuse the matter further, there can be a good deal of feedback between allergic and non-allergic illnesses, in both directions. Allergic symptoms can be exacerbated, or even provoked by other illnesses, as well as vice versa. This can make it hard to determine which problem is causing which.

Type A illnesses

These may be caused exclusively by Type A allergy, but sometimes Type B allergies and other factors play a part. In some types of eczema, for example, the underlying problem may be an allergy to dust mites, and this causes the itch. But the rash may not appear until the patient scratches the itch. Once the skin has been abraded by scratching, bacteria can easily set up an infection and this may lead to impetigo. There are also indirect influences on allergic illnesses. For instance, stress frequently aggravates eczema (dermatitis), partly because under such circumstances the itch becomes more irritating and the patient scratches more, and partly because stress changes the immune system's reaction to allergic triggers (see page 41). Trace nutrient deficiencies will affect most allergies, particularly eczema.

Food allergies and intolerances

Apart from eating certain foods very frequently, the factors that contribute to the development of Type B food allergy are not well understood. The role of gut flora (the bacteria and single-celled organisms that live inside our intestines) in food allergy and intolerance has received a lot of attention recently. There is evidence that levels of yeast such as Candida and of other organisms such as Giardia are important in irritable bowel syndrome and other disorders, and that severe digestive upsets – for instance, diarrhoea – can somehow weaken the gut and make it sensitive (see Chapter 4). Antibiotics taken to treat any infection may cause further problems: by killing off normal, healthy gut flora, they can clear the way for overgrowth of damaging organisms, leading to food intolerance.

ALLERGIES AND GENERAL HEALTH

Chapter 9 details the enormous variety of illnesses that allergies can cause or complicate, ranging from acne

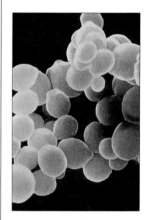

CANDIDA ALBICANS
Yeast micro-organisms like Candida albicans *are suspected of being involved in a range of Type B conditions, especially gastro-intestinal disorders.*

ITCHY FINGERS
Skin allergies often cause itchiness, and scratching, which breaks the skin and leaves it vulnerable to infection. Babies with eczema can be protected by swathing their hands in soft mittens, breaking this chain of events.

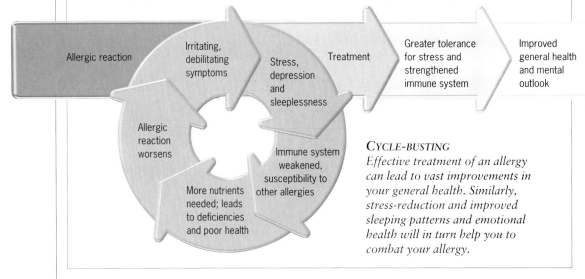

BREAKING THE CYCLE

An allergic reaction may cause mental and physical stress and set up a worsening cycle of weakened immunity and further allergic reactions. By controlling your symptoms you can break the cycle and improve your health.

Allergic reaction

Irritating, debilitating symptoms

Stress, depression and sleeplessness

Treatment

Greater tolerance for stress and strengthened immune system

Improved general health and mental outlook

Allergic reaction worsens

More nutrients needed; leads to deficiencies and poor health

Immune system weakened, susceptibility to other allergies

CYCLE-BUSTING
Effective treatment of an allergy can lead to vast improvements in your general health. Similarly, stress-reduction and improved sleeping patterns and emotional health will in turn help you to combat your allergy.

to infertility. But leaving the direct effects of allergic reactions to one side, what about their indirect effects? It is clear that many allergies can be chronic or recurrent in nature, which can have a two-fold effect.

First, with the immune system in a constant state of arousal, many of the body's disease-fighting resources will be diverted from more useful pursuits, and at the same time essential nutrients, such as zinc and magnesium, will be used up. Secondly, the chronic, irritating and debilitating nature of many allergic disorders must take its toll on the psychological health of the individual. As we shall see, the mind has a very real influence over the immune system, and untreated allergies and poor mental health can produce a negative feedback loop.

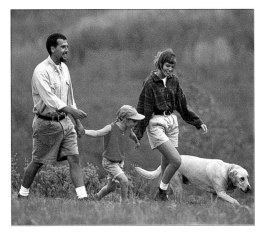

FREEDOM FROM ALLERGY MISERY
People who have suffered chronic ailments for decades can find that a few simple avoidance strategies can transform their lives, enabling them to do and enjoy things – from walking uphill to sleeping through the night – that were previously beyond them.

Negative feedback

If an allergy sufferer is depressed, stressed, irritable and losing sleep because of his or her condition, the immune system will suffer accordingly, and the patient's health will get worse. As the body becomes more vulnerable, so it becomes more susceptible to other allergens. Thus a dairy allergy that is left unchecked can lead to the development of sensitivities to other foodstuffs. As digestion suffers, so does nutrition, dealing another blow to health. Allergies make general health worse, which in turn worsens the allergies. This is negative feedback.

Breaking the cycle

Many sufferers of Type B allergies endure this sort of constant, grinding misery for years on end, which is why successful treatment can produce such remarkable effects. A careful elimination diet (see Chapters 2 and 4) can break this negative cycle, and provide dramatic health gains. The sufferer is relieved from what seemed to be an intractable problem, which doctors either would not take seriously, or could not treat. Many only realise how ill they were in retrospect. This sort of recovery starts its own positive feedback loop. Once a person's general health and positive mental outlook are restored, they may even be able to start eating some of the foodstuffs that used to trigger symptoms.

Protecting Against Allergy with

Nutrient Boosts

Many nutrients that are found widely in foods can help to protect you against allergies. To function at its best, your immune system needs all these nutrients and any deficiencies can make your system more prone to allergies.

There are some general rules about eating to reduce the risk of allergies. First you should vary your diet as widely as possible. Try not to eat wheat or milk products too often.

Limit the number of times a day you have tea, coffee, cola or soft drinks. Drink water more often, preferably bottled or filtered.

Include as many different vegetables and fruits as possible – try to have five good servings every day, in addition to potatoes. Use fresh food as much as possible to cut down on additives and choose organic foods when you can, especially for whole foods or if you mean to eat the skin.

Eat some oily fish or take some fish oil or linseed oil at least once or twice a week, but avoid fish oil if you are planning to conceive.

Use good quality oils from single sources (safflower, sunflower, olive) for dressings and cooking, and cut down on animal fat.

If you are vegetarian or vegan make sure you plan your diet to get a sufficient amount of protein.

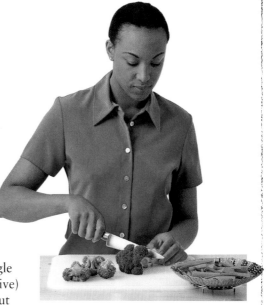

VEGETABLE NUTRIENT BOOST
A selection of steamed vegetables eaten every day can give a much needed boost to your immune system.

MEAL SUGGESTIONS

BREAKFAST

▶ *A bowl of porridge oats and soya milk, topped with banana.*

▶ *Rice cakes topped with a little hazel, almond or cashew nut butter and watermelon.*

LIGHT MEAL

▶ *Couscous salad with asparagus, cucumber and red onion.*

▶ *Turkey or prawn salad with a selection of leaves, cucumber, bean sprouts and boiled potatoes.*

MAIN MEAL

▶ *Roast guinea fowl or baked trout with a selection of steamed or roast vegetables.*

▶ *Baked mackerel with steamed green vegetables and assorted grains.*

DESSERT

▶ *Fresh fruit salad (can be accompanied by soya yoghurt).*

▶ *Pancakes made from lentil or millet flour served with a variety of hot or cold fillings.*

THE SPICE OF LIFE
Careful thought, fresh ingredients and variety are the keys to a healthy, low-allergen diet.

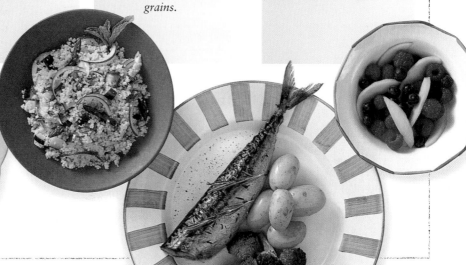

ALLERGY TESTING

Pinpointing allergens can be extremely difficult, and complicated by delayed effects, multiple allergies and false results. The practitioner's experience is a vital tool in accurate diagnosis.

The first step is to suspect allergy. Many people, including some doctors, have trouble with this, especially when foods are involved. The wider implications of allergies and intolerances are still not well understood or accepted by many in the medical profession. This means that if you suspect that you suffer from a nonstraightforward allergy, you may have to take the initiative in getting yourself referred and tested. Your doctor may be unaware of the full range of options available, so use this chapter as a very brief guide, and research the organisations and services available to you locally.

PRACTITIONERS

A practitioner's approach to diagnosis and testing will reflect his or her approach to the field as a whole. Immunologists, who restrict their focus to allergy Types I to IV, will only be interested in diagnostic methods which test immune response directly (such as measurement of specific antibodies), or in testing for a response that fits the classification (such as skin tests). Environmental allergists also use these methods, but

will look further afield. They will still want to base their diagnosis on a test with sound scientific principles, such as food challenges, or nutritional tests. Alternative practitioners advocate a range of methods, arguing that as long as a test works and suggests a useful treatment, it does not matter whether or not its mechanism is understood. This applies to tests like the auriculocardiac reflex, Vega testing or dowsing (see below).

The pros and cons of each approach

The immunological approach has several advantages. Testing is done in controlled situations, so it should be possible to replicate results. Also, since the underlying mechanisms are understood, these tests may provide a better rationale for devising treatment, or a better basis for research in the area. The drawbacks lie in the narrow focus of this approach, which only really works for Type I allergies, mostly ignoring Types II-IV, and Type B allergies. Also, even these 'scientific' tests do not give results as reliable as immunologists would like to believe.

The tests used by environmental allergists share some of these problems and may also involve a lot of effort. Alternative tests tend not to be supported by rigorous study, and it is hard to verify or assess the claims made for them on strictly scientific grounds.

Experience counts

Success in testing, in terms of finding the right treatment, depends on the skill and experience of the tester. Alternative tests like dowsing may reflect this, with the dowser's knowledge and experience causing slight movements that lead to diagnosis.

TESTS

Despite the wide range of tests available, there is one method which is generally agreed to provide firm diagnostic evidence,

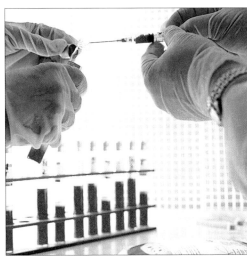

LAB TESTS
Controlled laboratory testing is a favoured diagnostic tool for conventional medicine for reasons of objectivity, reproducibility and reliability. Unfortunately few lab tests for allergies exist, and those that do, such as the blood test shown on the right, are limited in scope. Some have a high margin of error.

although it is laborious and inconvenient: the double-blind challenge. This test can be used for ingestants, as a food challenge, or for inhalants, as a vapour challenge. Skin testing is a sort of contact challenge.

Challenges

These involve presenting the patient with the suspect allergen to see whether it produces a reaction. If the test is positive several times in a row, it is unlikely to be a coincidence. Scientists, however, consider that results can only be trusted if the patient does not know which reaction to expect, so that he or she does not imagine or magnify the symptoms.

Double-blind

The solution is to do the challenges 'double-blind', so that neither the patient nor the doctor can influence the outcome by their various prejudices. The test substances are prepared by a third party, so that neither the patient nor the doctor know which is which and the patient may be presented with either a real test substance or a harmless control, known as a placebo. If a food is being tested, the challenge might come as a highly flavoured stew made with ingredients that are safe for that patient, with the suspect food blended in so that it is undetectable.

Problems

The whole process is laborious, expensive and time-consuming. A series of appointments is needed, and some challenges only cause symptoms slowly or when given repeatedly. In pioneer studies on hyperactivity and migraine at Great Ormond Street Hospital, and irritable bowel syndrome at Cambridge, each challenge had to be administered for two full weeks.

Elaborate double-blind procedures are necessary in rigorous scientific trials, but in practice most environmental allergists find that open food challenges give good enough results to prescribe successful treatments.

Synergistic factors

A major problem is the role of synergistic factors. These are external factors that aggravate intolerance – for instance, taking exercise, aspirin or alcohol, or being premenstrual. Combinations of certain foods can cause reactions, even when each food alone does not. If the relevant synergistic factor is absent, the challenge will be negative even though there is a genuine sensitivity – either an allergy or an intolerance.

This means that although double-blind challenges prove sensitivity when they are positive, they do not disprove it when negative. Sometimes this is not properly understood, and double-blind challenges are interpreted incorrectly to 'disprove' the possibility of sensitivity as a cause of illness.

Measurement of specific IgE antibodies (RAST)

Originally this test used radioactive isotopes and was called the radio-allergosorbent test (abbreviated to RAST). This test and its

Fast track
Normally food elimination diets and subsequent food challenges need to be done over several weeks, leaving plenty of time between each challenge. At special allergy treatment centres like the Airedale Allergy Centre in England, careful medical supervision allows patients to go on strict fasts which clear their systems of allergens. After such fasts, patients can then try several food challenges a day, helping to radically speed up identification of trigger foods and substances.

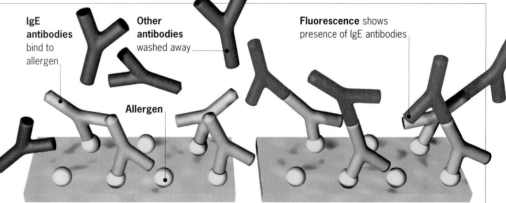

THE RAST TEST

The RAST test is widely accepted as the standard laboratory test for Type I allergies. Dishes or tubes precoated with specific allergens are used, and the test is now routine, easily performed and increasingly reliable. Nonetheless, it is far from perfect, and only limited in scope – for instance, it only tests for IgE antibodies, just one of the types involved in allergic reactions.

IgE antibodies bind to allergen

Other antibodies washed away

Allergen

Fluorescence shows presence of IgE antibodies

STEP 1
Allergens are attached to a dish and a sample of blood passed over them, then washed off. If IgE antibodies are present they bind to the allergens.

STEP 2
A special fluorescent antibody is then applied, which binds with any bound IgE antibody. Fluorescence shows the patient has antibodies specific to the test allergen.

The Conventional Allergist

Perhaps the first port of call for an allergy sufferer, after their GP, will be a conventional, or 'classical' allergist. The allergist will use the basic tools of conventional medicine to identify and help you to manage your allergy.

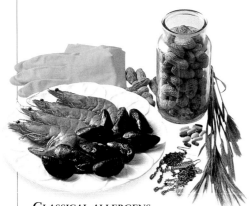

CLASSICAL ALLERGENS
Conventional allergists will consider the role of allergens like pollen, nickel, latex or common Type A food triggers (like nuts and shellfish). These are substances that provoke Type I allergic reactions. They are more likely to dismiss sources of allergen such as chemical fumes, caffeine or food additives.

Many sufferers feel let down by the failure of some practitioners to take any but the most straightforward allergies seriously. When GPs cannot find any obvious physical cause for vague, chronic symptoms they are more likely to make a diagnosis of stress or hypochondria than consider the role of allergy. So one of the first and most important things that an allergist provides is a sympathetic and believing ear.

What is an allergist?
The conventional allergist is a trained doctor. He or she will have been through medical school and done postgraduate training in general medicine and probably a related speciality such as ear, nose and throat or paediatrics. In the UK, most allergists will have then learned the job by apprenticeship, without a further diploma, but in the USA and most European countries they will also have a diploma in allergology.

What does a diploma in allergology cover?
A wide range of topics are covered, including relevant aspects of toxicology, immunology, nutrition, veterinary medicine, botany, zoology, microbiology, mycology (the study of fungi), food technology, chemistry and occupational hygiene. All of these disciplines are important for a proper understanding of the sources and nature of possible allergens and toxins.

How does the approach of an allergy specialist differ from that of a GP?
One of the biggest differences is the amount of time spent on the consultation, since few GP's can afford to devote an hour to every new patient, whereas most allergists do just that. The allergist is more aware of dangers in the environment and diet and also better informed in the use of diagnostic and treatment methods. He or she will often prefer to get to the root causes of the illness, rather than simply suppressing the symptoms.

Origins

During the 1960s two teams were searching for the immunoglobin involved in Type I allergic reactions. In 1967 the husband and wife team of Teruko and Kimishige Ishizaka described a new type of immunoglobin which they showed was involved in hay fever allergy – the IgE immunoglobin. In the same year Swedish researchers Johansson and Bennich described the same substance, and, together with L. Wide, developed a method for measuring levels of it in blood serum, using radioactive particles. This was the radio-allergosorbent test, or RAST for short.

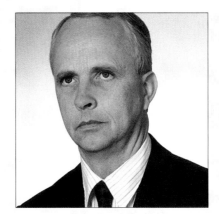

S. GUNNAR O. JOHANSSON
Together with his partner, Hans Bennich, Johansson identified IgE and developed the RAST test.

What can I expect at a consultation?

All allergy consultations start with a lengthy and detailed history, which can often take an hour or more. The doctor will wish to know minute details about the patient's diet, work and lifestyle, to see if any clues emerge. A patient may have a skin rash, for example, that first appeared a couple of months after a new washing powder was introduced, or have found that symptoms disappeared during a holiday in India, only to reappear on returning home. Once identified, avoidance of the causes (if possible) is often a matter of common sense. This is why talking is such an essential part of the allergist's procedure, and taking the time to listen to a patient can be excellent therapy in itself.

What sort of tests will the allergist carry out?

Sometimes the clues are so strong that the specialist stops there and advises a change of diet or lifestyle which might be completely successful. If not, the specialist may well do skin tests or blood tests to get more clues. Prick tests usually form the first line of testing, but in some cases, for reasons of safety,

blood tests such as RAST (see page 33) may be used. The patient may also be asked to keep an accurate diary of everything he or she eats and does, in the hope that unnoticed associations may emerge. If non-allergic conditions could be involved, the specialist will need to do a physical examination and may order various tests and X-rays.

What treatment might be offered?

Allergists with the appropriate expertise may use desensitisation, since it offers the possibility of attacking the root causes of the illness rather than simply suppressing

FINDING AN ALLERGIST

Registers of allergists in the UK are maintained by the two Learned Societies, which have confusingly similar names. The British Society for Allergy, Environmental and Nutritional Medicine (BSAENM) representing environmental allergists and clinical ecologists and The British Society for Allergy and Clinical Immunology (BSACI) for conventional allergists and immunologists. Most NHS allergists fall into the latter category or belong to both bodies and can be found by going through a GP.

The BSACI will supply a list of the allergy clinics nearest to you, and your doctor can get the names of local practitioners from the BSAENM (although they will not give the names of allergists directly to patients).

symptoms. In the UK, classic desensitisation was restricted in 1986, and now it is only used for insect-sting allergy and sometimes for hay fever. A few conventional allergists now use one of the newer forms of desensitisation (see Chapter 2), and this is gradually spreading as the evidence for their effectiveness gets stronger. The allergist also uses conventional drugs for conditions where avoidance and desensitisation are ineffective.

Basically the allergist's aim is to devise the best programme to help you to manage your allergy, integrating the various forms of conventional treatment available.

Will my GP refer me to an allergy specialist?

That depends first on whether the GP suspects allergy as a possible cause, and secondly, whether there are allergists locally to refer the patient to. Trained allergists are still rare in the UK, though not in North America or western Europe. In the UK, most patients who come to allergists report that they had to ask their GP for the referral, and in some cases even change their GP to get a referral.

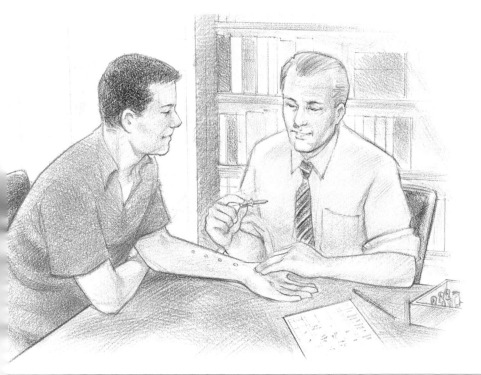

ALLERGY TESTING
The allergist may have a range of allergen samples (for example, pollen extracts) for skin prick testing. He will select the most likely allergens based on the pattern and history of symptoms.

Types of skin test

There are three main types of skin test – prick testing, intracutaneous (or intradermal testing) and patch testing. In prick testing, a tiny amount of allergen is introduced into the superficial layer of the skin. In intracutaneous testing, a larger quantity of allergen is injected directly into the dermis. Prick testing is more widely used, since it is easier, cheaper, less painful and has less chance of provoking a serious reaction. Intracutaneous tests are slightly more sensitive, and so may be done if a prick test does not give a clear result. Patch tests are used to test reactions to contact with the allergen, and involve attaching some of the test substance to the skin with a plaster to check for a wheal-and-flare response.

successors (which dispensed with the radio-active element but kept the name RAST) quickly became the standard 'blood test for allergies' in conventional medical circles. Its main advantage is that it gives a precise measurement of specific IgE antibodies in the blood. Its big disadvantage is that this is only of value with conditions caused by Type I allergy (see page 18). Unfortunately many doctors have adopted the view that if IgE antibody is not present, then there is no allergy. This is obviously flawed since it ignores the existence of the whole category of Type B allergies and allergy Types II-IV.

Skin tests

For many allergists the first line of physical investigation is skin testing. Tiny volumes of allergen, in liquid form, are introduced into the patient's skin. After 10 minutes or so, if there is specific IgE and if the mast cells are sensitive, the skin will blush red (flare) and produce a raised wheal due to the histamine released from those mast cells. This characteristic reaction is known as the wheal-and-flare response.

However, the skin mast cells in this particular person may not give the same reaction as those in the rest of the body. Also, skin tests are not always positive in cases of Type B allergy, although they can detect Type III and IV allergies if the skin is watched for long enough.

Tests of basophil and mast cell activation

Simple measurement of blood IgE says nothing about the state of the mast cells and basophils (see page 17), without which IgE cannot do any harm, however much there is. Hence these tests give a more realistic picture. Basophils are prepared from a blood sample and mixed with the allergen in a test tube. If there are IgE antibodies present, and if the basophils are susceptible to their effects, the latter undergo various cellular and biochemical changes which can be measured. For instance, when triggered by an allergen, the cell's contents may be released, in a process known as degranulation.

Dowsing

In this method, the practitioner holds a small pendulum over samples from the patient (blood, hair, etc.) and concentrates

> **WARNING**
> *Skin testing is potentially dangerous; very occasionally it can cause a severe allergic reaction such as asthma or anaphylaxis. It should only be carried out with due precautions by experienced doctors, or under their supervision.*

SKIN-PRICK TEST

Skin testing is one of the key elements in the allergist's diagnostic armoury. The prick test provides a quick, easy, relatively safe method of checking that IgE antibodies are present and reacting with the mast cells in the skin.

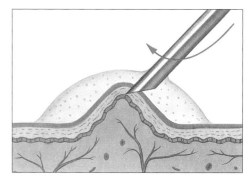

APPLICATION OF ALLERGEN EXTRACT
Usually, a small drop of extract is put on the forearm. Testing sites should be about 2 cm (1 in) apart, in two or three rows.

PRICKING THE SKIN
The allergist pricks through the drop into the outer skin and watches for the wheal-and-flare response to appear 10-15 minutes later.

on the substance in question. By 'reading' the movements of the pendulum he or she makes a diagnosis. Clairvoyant powers are offered as one explanation for the phenomenon. Practitioners of impeccable integrity – many of whom refuse to take payment for this work – report excellent clinical results, far better than the 60 per cent success rate that would be expected from lucky guesswork. Anecdotal evidence, however, is not the same as controlled studies.

Auriculocardiac reflex

This test is based on traditional Chinese medicine. Practitioners claim to be able to detect pulse alterations when the patient is exposed to substances to which he or she is thought to be 'allergic'.

Pulse rate changes

A more modern relation of this test was devised by American physician Dr Arthur Coca in the 1940s. An important figure in the early study of allergies, and one of the team who proposed the term atopy (see page 18), Coca claimed that challenging an allergic patient with a trigger food produced detectable changes in pulse rate. Many environmental allergists still use this test – in conjunction with others – but pulse changes are conventionally held to be unreliable.

Cytotoxic test

In this test white blood cells are taken from a blood sample and incubated with various substances and foodstuffs, after which a technician examines the specimens to see what damage has been sustained. Blood cells from different people seem to show different patterns of damage to the cells, and substances that cause damage to the cells (substances which are said to be cytotoxic) are deemed to be allergenic or toxic for that patient. This is probably the most convincing test for Type B allergies, but has a high rate of false positive and false negative results, so it is not a suitable basis for long-term diets without checking with appropriate food challenges.

Nutritional tests

Conventional biochemical tests can be used to assess depletion of vitamin and trace-element levels in the body that are caused by allergic illness. Dietary advice and supplements can be prescribed based on the

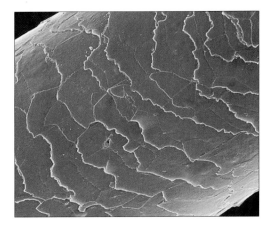

HAIR TESTING
Type B sufferers sometimes exhibit high levels of heavy metals (for example, lead, mercury, cadmium) which may be deposited in the hair. Strands of hair are thus often used in tests for heavy metals.

results. Most nutritional tests are carried out on blood samples, but urine and in some cases sweat may also be used where appropriate. Often the quality and results of these tests may depend simply on the laboratory carrying them out, making them unreliable in general.

Applied kinesiology

Also known as the 'muscle weakness test'. Practitioners claim that they can detect changes in muscle strength when the patient holds a glass phial containing a suspect allergen. The patient is said to be 'allergic' to the substances in bottles that caused his or her muscles to go weak. Theories involving bioelectromagnetism have been advanced to explain the phenomenon.

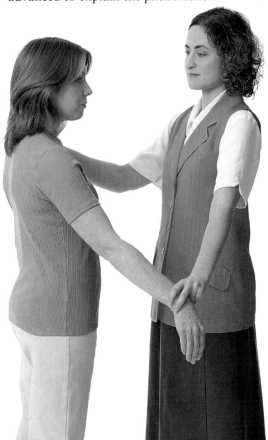

APPLIED KINESIOLOGY
A kinesiologist will attempt to detect fluctuations in muscle strength by pushing or resisting the patient's attempts to move. If the patient grows weaker when holding various substances, the kinesiologist will diagnose an allergy to that substance.

37

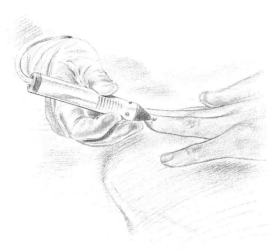

In expert hands this method seems to have a good success rate, and the allergens identified often correspond closely to those suggested by patients' histories, food challenges and conventional tests.

IgG ELISA testing

This is a new and relatively unproven development, but potentially offers the same degree of scientific rigour as IgE testing. It tests for the presence of IgG antibodies in the patient's blood. IgG is involved in Type II and III allergies, especially food allergies, where reactions are delayed. So this procedure might extend the range of conventional allergy testing to include a slightly wider variety of allergies.

Acupuncture and Vega testing

Acupuncturists claim that the electrical resistance of the skin varies, particularly around acupuncture points. Machines like the Vegatest exploit this property by measuring changes in skin conductivity when a vial containing 'allergen' is inserted into the circuit. If this happens the patient is deemed to be 'allergic'.

HOW EFFECTIVE ARE TESTS?

The fact that there are so many different tests for allergy is a warning that none of them is perfect. Even the best tests for allergies have significant error rates, and seem to have a limited applicability.

Conventional tests

RAST testing, basophil degranulation testing and skin testing have been assessed for accuracy in hay fever. This is a good disease to use for 'testing the tests', since the condition is usually clear-cut enough to make a diagnosis without tests. All three tests give correct results in about 80 per cent of cases, with false-positive and false-negative rates of around 10 per cent each. Thus the tests are fairly accurate in the one allergic condition for which tests are not needed.

Shortfalls

But these tests, which are viewed by many conventional doctors as the standard 'tests for allergy', are much less useful when it comes to food reactions, even Type I food reactions. For Type B allergies, for which a reliable test is urgently needed, they are virtually useless. The only reliable and reproducable method of diagnosing Type B allergy, which comes up to rigorous scientific criteria, is through double blind challenges (see page 33).

In general, allergists find that intelligent suggestions based on informed guesswork will have roughly a 60 per cent success rate. Treatments based on test diagnoses give a similar result. To properly assess which test is best, controlled trials are needed, but unfortunately these are not being done. As a result, many allergists rely on a process of trial-and-error, which remains the best option available.

WHAT TO DO IF TESTING IS INCONCLUSIVE

Allergy testing is never 100 per cent reliable. The best figures available indicate a total inaccuracy rate of 25 per cent – that is, each diagnosis has at least a 1:4 chance of being wrong. Some of the less conventional methods might give better results but there is no hard proof to back up their claims.

Allergists adopt various strategies to cope with this uncertainty. Some choose to pretend it doesn't exist: patients should be very careful of practitioners who claim an infallible test method. Responsible allergists either rely on guesswork, as explained above, or use tests of various types as a starting point for elimination trials. It should be remembered that all medical treatments are to some extent experiments, since the doctor never knows with absolute certainty that the treatment will work in a particular case. A doctor only feels happy that the diagnosis is right when the patient is cured – and even then he or she cannot be sure. To some extent all diagnoses are tentative, and in allergies this fact is made clearer than usual.

CHAPTER 2

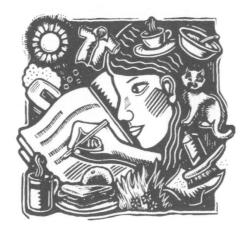

TREATING ALLERGIES

Different schools of allergists agree that the first line of defence against allergic illness is avoidance of the triggers. They also agree that stress and poor mental health can exacerbate and perhaps even cause many allergic symptoms, so comprehensive treatment must involve a mental perspective. Where the experts differ is over the form that more active treatment should take.

KEEPING ALLERGIES IN PERSPECTIVE

The power of the mind has long fascinated doctors. How much influence does the mind have on health? Allergy research suggests that psychological factors can influence allergic problems.

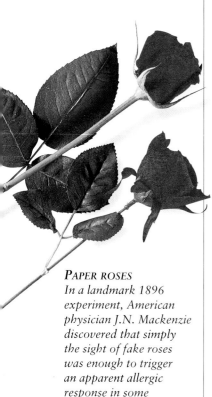

PAPER ROSES
In a landmark 1896 experiment, American physician J.N. Mackenzie discovered that simply the sight of fake roses was enough to trigger an apparent allergic response in some asthma sufferers.

At least 20 per cent of the UK population suffer from allergies, and there is a wide range of allergens – allergy producing substances – which cause allergic symptoms. People can react to an allergen in different ways. The reaction may be an immediate, acute response to an obvious allergen: for example, sneezing after exposure to grass pollen. Other reactions have delayed effects which are more difficult to spot because they have more general symptoms, such as headaches in response to a food. The cause of this type of delayed allergy is not always a single food or environmental allergen – it may be a combination of many different factors.

IS IT IN THE MIND?

An allergy specialist uses many different methods to identify the cause of a patient's allergic symptoms. The process involves a careful elimination of other causes that may produce allergy-like symptoms. Anxiety, depression and stress can produce the same physical symptoms as an allergy – tiredness, headaches, backache and indigestion for example. The allergist, therefore, needs to look at both the patient's physical and psychological history before deciding whether the symptoms are caused by an allergy or a psychological problem, or a combination of the two. A confusing factor is that stress and depression can themselves be caused by allergic reactions, so that allergies might be producing other symptoms indirectly.

The power of the mind

A hundred years ago, the American physician J.N. Mackenzie conducted a well-known experiment in which he provoked asthma attacks in people allergic to roses by using fake paper roses. In 1987 psychologist Harry Kotses added to these findings, when in a study of 30 normal people at Ohio University, he demonstrated that constriction of the airways (which happens in asthma) could also be provoked in normal individuals in response to suggestion.

In 1986, research from Hamburg confirmed the connection between a person's psychological state and his or her physical condition. Results from 44 asthma sufferers revealed that stress was capable of causing an asthma attack identical to one brought on by allergy, regardless of the severity of the subjects' actual allergies. It appears that, in some cases at least, the physical symptoms of allergy can be produced through psychological pressure.

Increased emotional sensitivity and allergy

The picture is further confused because some research suggests that allergic people have an increased emotional sensitivity – in other words they are more susceptible to anxiety or depression. Patients who are anxious or depressed are less likely to take their medication regularly, and hence their symptoms may get worse. This gives a confusing correlation between psychological problems and allergic conditions, where it is not clear if one is causing or influencing the other.

How can allergic and psychological causes be differentiated?

Obviously there is some degree of overlap between symptoms caused by allergy and those caused by psychological factors, so how do you tell them apart? There is no simple answer. An individual allergist's method of diagnosis depends on his or her approach and careful interpretation of the patient's medical history. Allergists will usually wait until they see the results of treatment before they decide about the main cause of symptoms, but either way, the fact that symptoms are linked with stress does not necessarily exclude an allergic cause.

STRESS AND ALLERGY

Your emotional state or response to stress can modify your ability to cope with infection, cancer, allergens and autoimmune diseases. The study of how this happens is a fast developing research field called neuroimmunology. Several studies have shown that stress can change both the production of antibodies and the function of white cells, usually resulting in suppression of the immune system. Paradoxically this may actually worsen allergic reactions.

Examples of acute allergic symptoms resulting from acute stress are 'World cup' and 'earthquake' urticaria (nettle rash), where the stress induced by these events has led to outbreaks of allergic skin reactions. In fact research from Japan has suggested that all chronic urticaria involves a combination of physical and psychological causes. This is not the same as saying that stress alone can cause symptoms – in some instances this may be the case, but in others stress will only cause symptoms if an allergy already exists.

The other side of the coin is that allergic conditions can cause stress. For example, attention deficit disorder in children can cause extreme tensions within families.

Minimising the effects of stress

It is your own response to stress that determines the effect that it has on your health. When dealt with properly, stress can actually be beneficial rather than harmful. The practical steps you need to take when dealing with stress are: first, identify the situations that you find particularly stressful; second, notice how this makes you feel; and third, put into action an immediate stress intervention programme (see page 51).

Research has shown that people with an extrovert personality, or those who are humorous, creative or strong-willed, are more likely to have a strong immune system, as these people tend to deal positively with stress. Sleeping well can also reduce stress levels and enhance your immune system.

What stress management can achieve

Some asthma sufferers can be significantly helped by psychological therapies: doctors from Boston discovered that stress management programmes helped children with asthma to carry out daily activities with reduced breathing difficulties, and more easily than those in a control group who had not undergone the programmes.

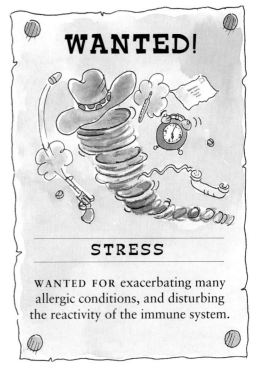

WANTED FOR exacerbating many allergic conditions, and disturbing the reactivity of the immune system.

STRESS AND THE IMMUNE SYSTEM

Stress interacts with the immune system in a complex fashion. When under stress, the brain triggers the release of hormones from hormone production centres like the hypothalamus, and chemical messengers from the nerves. These act in concert to affect the cells of the immune system, increasing both the likelihood of initial sensitisation – developing an allergy in the first place – and the likelihood of subsequent reactions, and also increasing the severity of reactions. These reactions can then feed back, causing more stress by producing allergic reactions, and acting directly on the brain to increase arousal and neural activity.

| Stress | → | Hormone production altered and chemical messengers produced by the nerves are changed | → | These changes affect the cells of the immune system | → | Likelihood of initial sensitisation increases; threshold for provoking allergic reaction lowered and severity of reaction increased |

HOW DOCTORS MANAGE ALLERGY

The first step in the conventional treatment of allergies is avoidance. When this is not possible doctors may then use drugs, and some may use immunotherapy.

Avoiding allergens can be achieved in two ways: either by changing your habits to avoid the environment where the allergens are found, or by changing your environment to remove the allergens. Evidence suggests that exposure to allergens early in life may be the number one trigger for development of allergy. This means that the best time to start preventing allergies is during pregnancy and the first year of a child's life. This is especially so if one or both parents are sufferers, as allergies are to some degree hereditary and their child will be at more risk of developing one.

Reducing early exposure

There are a number of findings that provide valuable direction for parents looking to safeguard their children against allergies and asthma. Preliminary research suggests that avoiding potentially reactive food (food that the parents might be allergic to) may be important even in the first half of pregnancy. The period of particular susceptibility to sensitisation is thought to be relatively short – lasting up to six months after birth. Studies have shown that infants who are at risk of developing allergy because their parents are allergic have less eczema and food allergy if their mothers avoid allergic foods in late pregnancy and during breastfeeding. Some protein from substances ingested by the mother is secreted unchanged in breast milk and this could sensitise the child to that

allergen. Avoiding the common allergens (milk, fish, nuts, soya, wheat and oranges) until age 12 months can reduce the incidence of allergies among infants at risk. In one study at St Mary's Hospital on the Isle of Wight, 40 per cent of the 'at risk' infants observed who were not on a special diet developed allergy, compared with only 13 per cent of those who avoided the common allergens. Exposure to pets (especially cats) during the child's first year of life also appears to be an important factor in the development of hypersensitivity. Lastly, parental smoking has been shown to have a profound effect on the prevalence of asthma and allergies in children.

AVOIDING ENVIRONMENTAL TRIGGERS

Environmental allergies are caused by substances that are found in the air or immediate environment and can be either seasonal, such as hay fever, or perennial – allergies that continue throughout the year – such as asthma. Identification is the first vital step in avoidance, and clues such as when and where symptoms come on can help.

If, for instance, the allergy is seasonal, it is most likely caused by pollens or seasonal mould spores. Avoiding mould and pollens is difficult, although hay fever sufferers can try to stay indoors and away from fields at the height of the season.

If symptoms improve or worsen depending on location, then you should suspect either indoor or outdoor pollutants as appropriate. Sulphur dioxide, nitrogen dioxide and ozone from vehicle or industrial exhausts are likely outdoor culprits. Within the home and office, cigarette smoke and perfumed products are common suspects.

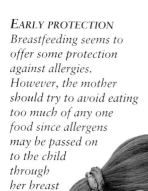

EARLY PROTECTION
Breastfeeding seems to offer some protection against allergies. However, the mother should try to avoid eating too much of any one food since allergens may be passed on to the child through her breast milk.

Dust mites and pets

The house dust mite is the most common allergen to trigger allergic asthma and rhinitis, while allergies to pet dander (flakes of skin), hair, saliva and urine are among the most common forms of allergy suffered today. Preventative measures like special vacuum cleaners, special mattress covers, hot washing, removing carpets and using air filters can all help (see Chapter 3).

AVOIDING FOOD TRIGGERS

Food reactions can be either immediate or delayed (see Chapter 4). Immediate reactions are obvious – they trigger symptoms such as itching and swelling around the mouth within minutes of contact – and the only proven treatment is strict avoidance of the offending food. Some allergies, in particular peanut allergy, can cause anaphylaxis (see Chapter 7), and sufferers should always carry adrenaline in case of exposure.

Hidden food allergy occurs when the body does not react immediately, or obviously to a food. Common symptoms include migraine, irritable bowel syndrome and fatigue. Hidden food allergies are also treated by avoiding the offending foods, although identifying the triggers may be difficult. A diet-and-symptom diary can help to provide some pointers (see page 44). Unfortunately symptoms of hidden food allergy will rarely be caused solely by a reaction to one food and avoidance of a single food may not solve the problem.

Identifying the culprits

Some conditions are often associated with a particular food, for instance wheat with irritable bowel syndrome. Avoiding these foods for two weeks may help with identification, but this only succeeds in a few cases. Constant craving for a particular food, often a sign of 'addiction', may also indicate an allergy, but a definite diagnosis may only be reached with a formal elimination diet.

The elimination diet

An elimination diet needs to be tried for one to three weeks. This means leaving out potentially allergenic foods until the body has had a chance to stop reacting to them. The foods are then reintroduced one by one and sensitivity to a food should become obvious, as symptoms will recur. An elimination diet should never be tried during

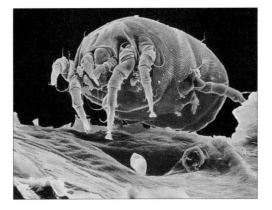

pregnancy or acute viral illness, and prescription medications should be continued throughout the diet, unless your doctor has advised otherwise. Non-essential medication, on the other hand, should be avoided.

The tolerated foods diet

After problem foods have been identified they can be avoided, leaving only tolerated foods in your daily diet. It is very important when embarking on elimination diets and tolerated foods diets to enlist the help of a dietitian: excluding foods can result in a nutritionally inadequate diet. You may find that after a period you can tolerate the problem foods again.

NUTRITION AND ALLERGY

Patients with allergic conditions are often deficient in zinc and magnesium, and some allergists recommend supplements. Zinc deficiency has been associated with hyperactivity, and low magnesium intake may be involved in asthma. These deficiencies are on the increase, possibly due to a wide-

DUST MITE
Although impossible to see with the naked eye, this tiny spider-like insect can cause and exacerbate asthma attacks and other symptoms. Regular washing of bedding and vacuuming of mattresses and upholstery can help to lessen the problem.

DIETARY DEFENCE
A diet rich in vitamins and trace minerals can help to alleviate the symptoms of allergic attacks. These are found especially in green vegetables, fruit, meat, fish and whole grains.

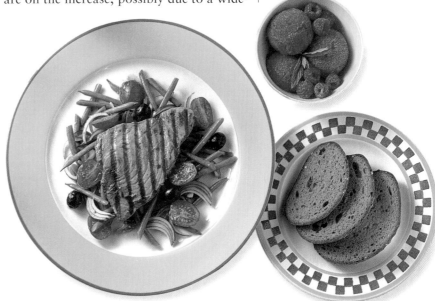

Identifying Your Allergy with an

Allergy Diary

It is easy to lose track of how symptoms change from day to day, or even from hour to hour. An allergy diary is an essential tool for helping you to identify which foods or environmental exposures are causing your symptoms.

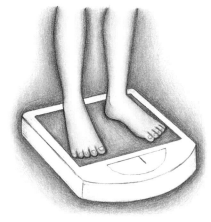

WEIGHING THE EVIDENCE
Record your weight every night after going to the toilet. A sudden gain in weight is a sign of water retention – a common food reaction.

Allergies can be difficult to identify but keeping an allergy diary is a simple first step in the investigation process that can yield some interesting results. Accuracy is essential in order to build up a clear picture of what could be triggering your symptoms. Simple food allergies may become clear by eliminating suspect foods and recording the results. Hidden food allergies are much harder to detect. It may help to keep a supplementary chart listing all the food you have eaten each day for a week. Count how many times a day you eat each food (this type of allergy is usually to a frequently eaten food).

Conclusively relating your symptoms to your diet will be difficult – you may need to do an elimination diet (see page 43).

WEEKLY ALLERGY CHART

The chart below shows you the information you need to record to help you to expose an allergy and its triggers. It needs to be completed regularly, at least once a day and more often if possible. Remember to record any current medication which you take for your allergies or for any other symptom – you could be reacting to one of these.

	MONDAY	TUESDAY	WEDNESDAY
Symptoms (e.g. Headache)	Migraine	Diarrhoea, migraine	No symptoms
Severity (on a scale of 1-5)	4	3 and 2	–
Weight at night	60 kg 133 lbs	60.5 kg 134 lbs	60 kg 133 lbs
Medications	Aspirin	Loperamide	None
Locations during day	Home Office	Home Office	Day off (stayed home)
Activities	Cooking, cleaning, working at desk	Cooking, working at desk, photocopying	Cooking, Gardening
Any unusual foods eaten	None	None	Nuts
Notes	Migraine came on in evening	Photocopier smelled strongly	Felt better

INTERPRETING YOUR CHARTS

After a week or two of keeping your charts, start a series of comparisons to see if there is a pattern to your symptoms and to help you to determine any possible triggers. Compare charts from days when you felt ill with days when you felt well and try to spot the differences in the foods that you ate and the activities you carried out. Certain tasks may provoke an allergic reaction immediately or later, even the next day. This may indicate that they bring you into contact with an allergen, or that they are a source of stress. Armed with a list of suspects from your allergy diary, you and your doctor will have a much better chance of identifying the substances which are making you ill, and avoiding or treating them more successfully.

COMMON ANTIHISTAMINES

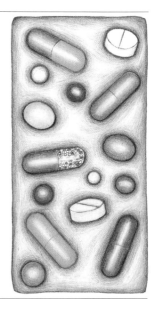

DRUG	EFFECT
Terfenidine	Widely used but can have a rare side effect – causing heart arrhythmia (irregular beating of the heart). Interaction with certain other drugs increases the chances of this, so a doctor or pharmacist should be consulted if you are using any other type of medication.
Astemizole	Slow onset of effect and stays in the body for up to four weeks after the last dose. Its absorption is delayed by food. It can also increase the risk of cardiac arrhythmia. Can cause increased appetite and weight gain.
Cetirizine, Loratidine and Acrivastine	All have been shown to be effective without any major problems (so long as patients keep to the recommended doses). Cetirizine may have extra benefits in seasonal asthma and urticaria.
Ketotifen	Produces additional benefits in children's coughs related to asthma. Can cause increased appetite and weight gain.

Warning All of these drugs must be avoided during pregnancy, especially during the first 14 weeks.

spread change in eating habits. Another dietary factor in asthma may be low levels of B vitamins and vitamin C. Large doses of these vitamins can reduce the allergic reaction of asthmatics to the inhalation of allergens, and B vitamins and antioxidants protect against the effects of stress. While supplements may help (taken under the guidance of a dietitian or doctor), particularly for people with special needs (such as pregnant women, teenagers or the elderly), a good diet is also essential.

CORTICOSTEROIDS

These drugs have an anti-inflammatory and immunosuppressive effect. They work by decreasing the body's production of cytokines – important chemical messengers that excite and activate elements of the immune system. Corticosteroids also decrease histamine release.

Local corticosteroids

Corticosteroid nasal drops and water-based nasal sprays are effective in controlling the nasal symptoms of hay fever and year-round allergic nasal congestion. They work by reducing inflammation and swelling in the lining of the nose.

Corticosteroids are also important in the control of asthma. Low doses are inhaled as a preventative medicine, and, taken every day, they can act to reduce inflammation of the airways and mucus production. Side effects are rare at low doses, but include hoarseness and a higher risk of thrush infections in the throat.

High doses for acute relief

Corticosteroids taken by mouth or injection are used to relieve very severe allergy symptoms. Short courses of oral steroids at higher doses are often needed for acute asthma. Prolonged treatment should be avoided if possible because of long-term side effects including rounding of the face, osteoporosis, raised blood pressure and many others.

ANTIHISTAMINES

Many of the symptoms of allergic disease are caused by the release of histamine. Antihistamine medications are therefore an important method of relieving these symptoms. They are effective for sneezing, itching, running noses and swelling, but they have little effect on nasal blockage.

There are two main groups of antihistamine. The older ones ('classical type') often cause unwanted side effects – sedation and

continued on page 48

WARNING

New research by the Medicines Control Agency shows that drinking grapefruit juice can be very dangerous or even lethal for people taking some antihistamines. Grapefruit juice contains high concentrations of a psoralen, a substance which acts to increase the concentration of these drugs in the bloodstream, causing inadvertent overdose.

Disodium cromoglycate

An alternative to steroidal medication is disodium cromoglycate which prevents the release of histamine from mast cells. It is safer but less effective than local corticosteroids, and the inhaled form is especially used for children.

Although it is not effective in all cases, for some patients capsules can successfully prevent a reaction to food. Take six to eight capsules 15 minutes before the meal. Swill them round the mouth with a little water, or chew them, before swallowing. Though apparently free of side effects it is only effective for short periods (a couple of hours). Sometimes patients are advised to take them regularly – if on holiday, for instance – at a lower dose: three to four before each meal.

The Environmental Allergist

Falling between conventional allergists and alternative practitioners, environmental allergists try to identify the causes of chronic symptoms and improve the recognition and management of allergic diseases.

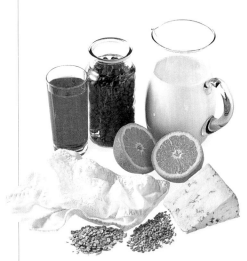

ENVIRONMENTAL ALLERGENS
These include all the substances recognised by conventional allergists – house dust, pollen, nickel, latex and many more – together with a wide range of environmental and dietary substances that conventional allergists dismiss.

ENVIRONMENTAL OR CONVENTIONAL?

The difference between the two branches of allergists is rooted in the origins of allergy as a branch of medicine, since which time conventional allergists (and the rest of mainstream practice) have taken the line that allergies are only present when there are measurable levels of IgE antibodies in the blood. This effectively excludes all delayed and hidden food allergy and many environmental allergies. Environmental allergists place more emphasis on the symptoms and, crucially, finding the causes of symptoms. This means that they treat a variety of conditions which conventional allergists consider to be psychosomatic.

The therapy offered by an environmental allergist (known as environmental medicine) aims to identify and reduce exposure to the environmental allergens that cause allergic reactions. These reactions can be caused by anything that is eaten, drunk, breathed or touched, irrespective of whether or not an immune response has been shown to be involved.

What qualifications and training do environmental allergists have?

Environmental allergists are qualified doctors who have had postgraduate training in either primary care medicine or another speciality. Most will have had further experience in allergy or immunology. In the UK the therapist should be a member of the British Society for Allergy, Environmental and Nutritional Medicine.

Who can benefit from environmental medicine?

The patients who will benefit most from environmental allergy treatment are those with chronic (long standing) health problems for which conventional medicine has found no explanation. Type B allergies typically fall into this pattern, with classic symptoms like tiredness, rhinitis, sinusitis, irritable bowel syndrome, headaches, chronic asthma, recurrent rashes or depression. Many of these patients are simply allergic to one or more environmental allergens but have not been recognised as allergy sufferers.

All of these symptoms need proper medical evaluation to exclude a possible non-allergic cause. In most cases, however, the patient will already have gone through detailed investigations which have turned up nothing, and their GP or conventional specialist will have blamed the condition on stress or hypochondria. Basically, any chronic symptoms whose cause has not been discovered will be of interest to the environmental physician.

Who can't benefit from environmental medicine?

Patients whose symptoms are due to a definite non-allergic cause, for example a virus or tumour or physical trauma, are not appropriate subjects for environmental allergy therapy. But allergic and non-allergic symptoms can coexist in the same patient, which confuses the issue.

How much scientific evidence is there for environmental medicine?

The British Society for Allergy, Environmental and Nutritional Medicine has published two documents on the standards of care and management for the allergy patient called *Effective Allergy Practice* and *Effective Nutritional*

Medicine, together with a text book on environmental medicine in clinical practice for doctors interested in the field. Between them these documents list nearly 500 references to research done in this field. Some traditional allergists are still critical of this evidence (for instance the Royal College of Physicians, in their 1990 report on allergy), but champions of the field claim that these criticisms are unfair, and that conventional allergists simply discount any research in environmental medicine, irrespective of its quality.

What happens in a session?

The allergist will take a very detailed clinical history, asking you about every symptom, its accurate chronology and the circumstances during or after which it occurred. He or she will also want to know about your health, history and lifestyle and what medications or alternative therapies you have tried.

PATCH TESTS
The therapist may perform some patch tests at the clinic, or demonstrate how they are done, so that you can do them yourself at home.

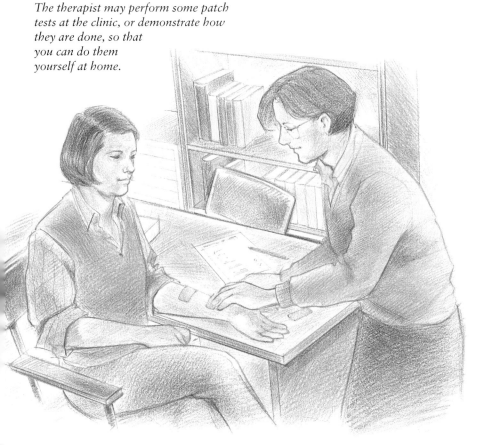

What sort of tests will the environmental allergist use?

Depending on the circumstances the allergist may do a full clinical examination and blood tests looking at the levels of immunoglobins and white blood cells (in other words, the main elements of the immune system), and possibly for important biochemical information, such as the levels of toxins and enzymes, or the presence of vitamin deficiencies. The allergist may try skin tests and will be prepared for a delayed reaction.

By examining your history, the allergist may identify some likely environmental or food culprits. Using this as a starting point, you can begin a programme of cleaning up your environment at home or an elimination diet, dealing with the most likely allergens first. You will be asked to keep a careful diary of events and foods. The suspect substances will then be reintroduced to you one by one to identify the triggers causing your symptoms.

What treatment will an environmental allergist offer?

Avoidance measures will be the first line of treatment, and the allergist will be able to offer guidelines, hints and tips. Whether or not a food allergy is suspected, nutritional factors will be discussed, and some dietary advice and possibly supplements offered. If a food has been identified as the allergen, the allergist will help you to plan a diet that you can tolerate. This diet will be individually tailored to compensate for any nutrients that you might miss out on through avoiding particular foods.

Based on the results of your skin tests and exclusion diet, the allergist may recommend a course of immunotherapy to desensitise your system to the allergens.

The aim of environmental treatment is to prevent provocation of symptoms and improve nutrition so that your health improves and you can enjoy life again.

WHAT YOU CAN DO AT HOME

Apart from clinic-based tests and immunotherapy injections, most of the steps involved in treating an allergy must be taken by you at home. There are two stages to this process: identification of the allergen and treatment. While trying to identify an allergen you can help the allergist by keeping an allergy diary (see page 44), and trying to observe associations between your health and various environmental factors.

During treatment of your allergy, make sure you follow all the avoidance measures you can manage, and all the dietary advice given. You should also take steps to reduce your stress levels. Take more exercise (but discuss what type with the allergist), learn some relaxation techniques, get more sleep and try some calming complementary measures, like Bach flower remedies or aromatherapy.

dry mouth – and cannot be used with other drugs such as sleeping tablets and anti-depressants. The newer, 'selective' histamine blockers rarely impair alertness (when they are taken at low doses) and do not generally have side effects when combined with alcohol or tranquillisers.

DESENSITISATION

If the allergen cannot be avoided, there is another form of treatment that offers a potential cure – immunotherapy, or desensitisation. This treatment aims to tackle the root cause of allergy by slowly encouraging the immune system to become less sensitive to the offending allergen, in other words desensitising it. There are currently three types of immunotherapy available: incremental dose allergen injection immunotherapy (IIT), and two low-dose methods – neutralisation and enzyme potentiated desensitisation (EPD).

Incremental dose allergen injection immunotherapy

This form of immunotherapy involves injecting the patient with doses of allergen – small enough not to produce an immune reaction at first, and gradually getting larger until the immune system can handle a 'normal' dose (such as one would find in the environment).

IIT has been proven to be effective in the treatment of insect sting allergies, hay fever, rhinitis and asthma. However, there is a major drawback, namely that up to 40 per cent of those treated will experience unpleasant and sometimes severe side effects, including anaphylaxis (see Chapter 7) – the degree of risk depends on the subject's health. Severe asthmatics and other vulnerable groups (people with heart disease for instance) should avoid such treatment. Until the mid 1980s IIT was popular, but the high rate of reactions and even deaths led to its use in the UK being restricted to a few specialised hospital allergy clinics.

Neutralisation

Neutralisation uses very low doses, self-administered on a regular basis. Patients are tested with mini-injections of allergen at gradually decreasing concentrations to determine the first dose that provokes no localised skin reaction. This is designated the neutralising dose – the strength of dose which is just adequate to 'neutralise' the allergic symptoms, but without causing any harmful side effects. This dose is then given regularly either by injection (two or three times a week) or by drops under the tongue (twice a day). A course continues for months or years – until the patient develops tolerance.

Trials of neutralisation – also known as low dose immunotherapy, or LDI – have shown it to be of benefit in allergic rhinitis, animal dander-induced asthma and food allergies. In contrast to the higher dose IIT, this method is reported to give immediate symptom relief and is apparently relatively free from severe or generalised reactions. There have been few reports of even mild reaction and this is in spite of the fact that it is regularly used by over 2000 doctors in the United States. Neutralisation is the preferred method of three out of four American allergy associations. The only area where IIT is still preferred is in the treatment of insect-sting allergies.

The neutralisation technique has been validated by double blind randomised trials showing its effectiveness in relieving and preventing symptoms of allergy. It should not be muddled with unproven techniques such as the provocation of symptoms by food extracts, or folk remedies like honey made from flowers with allergenic pollen.

Enzyme potentiated desensitisation

This is based on the discovery that a single, low dose of allergen can be 'potentiated' by being administered together with an enzyme called beta glucuronidase. Potentiation is where the enzyme somehow acts to make the allergen appear different to the immune system, so that tolerance develops instead of sensitisation and adverse reactions.

Clinical trials have shown that one to three doses of EPD per year can successfully treat hay fever, food allergy, ulcerative colitis and hyperactivity (see Chapter 8) with few side effects. EPD would thus appear to be a powerful and safe method for the treatment of clinical allergies.

There is still some scepticism about both low-dose methods – a 1992 Royal College of Physicians report concluded that large-scale trials are still needed. But all the evidence indicates that low-dose methods have fewer side effects and are safer than IIT.

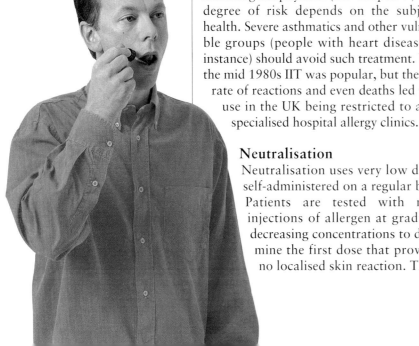

NEUTRALISATION
Neutralisation treatment may involve either injections or the administration of drops placed under the tongue. Once you have been tested to find your therapeutic dose, you will be able to treat yourself at home.

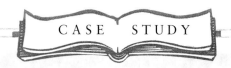

Multiple Allergy Sufferer

There are many allergens in the urban environment which can be inhaled, and many potentially allergy-causing foods. All of them can cause problems for rhinitis and asthma sufferers. When more than one allergic response is triggered the effect on the body can be most distressing and the symptoms can interfere with home and working life.

Robert is a 29-year-old office worker who has suffered from persistent cold symptoms since he was a teenager. Recently these symptoms have become worse and he has developed a dry throat, headache and eye irritation. At work his office is air conditioned, and he has a computer on his desk with a photocopier nearby. He and his wife have a cat. He eats well and is particularly fond of cheese and yoghurt.

Robert's GP tried a number of conventional treatments, but decongestants and antibiotics only produced a slight improvement. Eventually the doctor asked Robert about his medical history and decided to refer him to an allergy specialist.

WHAT SHOULD ROBERT DO?

Robert needs a practitioner who will consider all the details of his medical history. Whereas a GP may not have the time for this, an allergy specialist is trained to pick up on minor clues. The specialist should note that Robert's symptoms are continuous, making dust mites, mould spores, cat hairs or foods the most likely suspect allergens. The allergist should also note that Robert has a lot of dairy products in his diet and should do skin prick tests to check if he is allergic to cat hairs, spores, dust mites or other suspects. The allergist will then be able to give advice on how to avoid allergens to minimise the effects of these allergies, and how to find out whether foods are contributing.

Action Plan

DIET
Reduce intake of dairy products. Try a completely dairy food-free diet for three weeks if possible.

WORK
Improve ventilation in the office, getting more fresh air if possible. Sit away from photocopiers and get a radiation screen for the computer.

LIFESTYLE
Keep the cat out of the bedroom and living room (vacuum and damp dust these rooms). Try a course of neutralisation immunotherapy with cat allergen.

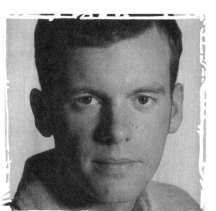

DIET
Milk and other dairy products are among the most common food allergens.

WORK
Air conditioning, computer screen glare and photocopier fumes can cause reactions in the eyes and the nasal lining.

LIFESTYLE
Daily exposure to pet hairs can sensitise people to allergens on them, or aggravate symptoms for someone who is already sensitised.

HOW THINGS TURNED OUT FOR ROBERT

The skin prick tests showed that Robert was allergic to cat hair. After following the specialist's advice on avoiding cat hair and other allergens Robert noticed a steady improvement in his symptoms. A dairy food-free diet produced definite results but Robert found it too difficult to cut out cheese and yoghurt and occasionally eats them as a treat. Further improvement followed a course of cat allergen immunotherapy.

ALTERNATIVE TREATMENTS

Conventional definitions of and treatments for allergies are limited to a narrow range of disorders. As a result, many people with chronic symptoms turn to alternative medicine for help.

Alternative medicine does not always lend itself to being tested in the same way as traditional medicines, because many of the conditions it treats are ill defined and treatments are often tailored to the individual. This makes it very difficult to prove that the treatments are effective. Because of this lack of proof, many doctors maintain that patients are vulnerable to therapists who claim to be able to provide a 'quick fix'. Nonetheless, patients are attracted by alternative medicine's holistic approach, considering the patient's body and mind as whole, and its gentler, more natural and less invasive techniques.

HERBAL REMEDIES

These have long been available for allergies. There is little scientific evidence that they work, but this does not mean that they are ineffective – rather that clinical trials have not been done. However, in 1992 a trial was done at Great Ormond Street Hospital, using traditional Chinese medicinal plants to treat atopic eczema in 37 children aged 1 to 18. The results showed a decrease in skin inflammation following use of a herbal remedy, with no short-term toxic effects. A further trial applying the same treatment to 40 adults gave similarly effective results.

Since then, however, concerns have been raised about the toxic effect of the treatments on the liver. Also, it seems likely that the benefits of these treatments arise from the direct anti-inflammatory effect of some ingredient contained within the herbs, acting like a conventional drug. This suggests that in some ways herbal remedies are similar to conventional drugs, whose side effects are better known and understood.

There is a national institute of medical herbalists: a qualified practitioner is designated MNIMH. They maintain that plant medicines have low toxicity and side effects and that they provide more balanced and safer remedies.

HOMEOPATHY

Invented by the German physician Samuel Hahnemann in the late 18th century, homeopathy is based on the principle that tiny amounts of the substance that causes an illness can be used to treat it. This may sound similar to immunotherapy, but in practice a homeopath uses such dilute quantities of the remedies that the patient may be given a solution which does not contain a single molecule of the original allergen.

Although scientists do not understand how this can work, some very careful studies show the effectiveness of homeopathy over a placebo (a fake solution with no therapeutic value), even in double-blind conditions (see page 33). A study by Dr David Reilly at the University of Glasgow showed that a homeopathic remedy using house dust mite allergen produced significant improvement in nine out of eleven asthma sufferers. There have been successful trials with hay fever as well.

To ensure that accurate treatment is received, a trained and qualified homeopath should be consulted. In the UK the Society of Homeopaths has a register of professionally trained practitioners.

STRESS RELIEF AND MIND THERAPIES

Many of the benefits of these therapies derive directly from their relaxing and stress-relieving effects. Stress, illness and the

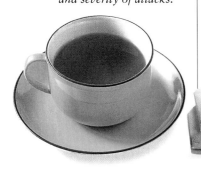

FENUGREEK TEA
As a digestive tonic, a cup of fenugreek tea drunk two to three times a day may be able to help to relieve symptoms of irritable bowel syndrome and reduce the frequency and severity of attacks.

Beating Stress-Related Asthma with

Meditation

It is well known that asthma attacks can be provoked by both acute and chronic stress. Meditation is an effective way to reduce the consequences of that stress and can calm your breathing, making attacks less likely in the first place.

Before you begin meditating make sure that you are in a warm and comfortable environment and that you will not be disturbed for at least half an hour.

Deep breathing

When you are comfortable start breathing more deeply than normal into your abdomen, and then let the breath exhale naturally and slowly. Breathe as slowly and deeply as you can, allowing the breath to push out your stomach as you breath in. Try not to let your upper chest or abdominal muscles become tense during this exercise. If you simply focus on your breathing then the rest of your body will naturally relax.

Repeating a mantra

Once you are relaxed you are ready to start the meditation. This is done by mentally repeating a 'mantra' – a specific word – on each outward breath. Monosyllabic words such as 'peace' may help the feeling of relaxation, but you can choose any word you like – the mantra helps to focus the mind. Try to keep this up for 10 minutes initially: stop if you start feeling restless and distracted.

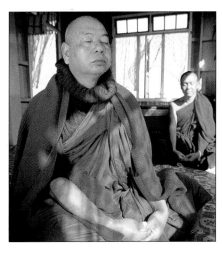

MEDITATION MASTERS
Since the 1st millennium BC followers of the Buddhist faith have used meditation to clear their minds and create a calm emotional state. Meditation has been found to help to boost the immune system and stave off allergic attacks.

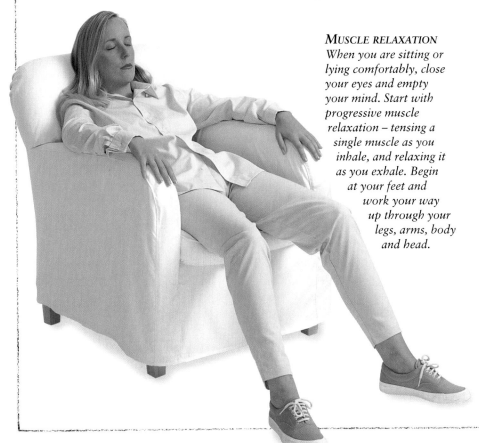

MUSCLE RELAXATION
When you are sitting or lying comfortably, close your eyes and empty your mind. Start with progressive muscle relaxation – tensing a single muscle as you inhale, and relaxing it as you exhale. Begin at your feet and work your way up through your legs, arms, body and head.

PRACTISE FOR PERFECTION

A few simple guides will help you to maintain your meditation regime. Each day set aside about 15 minutes at a regular time. Don't allow yourself to be distracted: disconnect the phone and find a quiet, comfortable place. The aim is to minimise your mind's attention on external elements. With practice you should be able to achieve longer periods with more benefit. If you find it difficult to meditate on your own, consider buying a cassette tape or finding a teacher of meditation. A yoga or t'ai chi teacher could also help you as meditation is part of both disciplines.

state of the immune system are intimately connected (see page 41), and just as psychological factors can cause or exacerbate some allergic illnesses, mind therapies can often help to treat them.

These therapies take two main forms. First, there are relaxation techniques, which include physical therapies such as yoga and massage, together with deep-breathing techniques and meditation. Second, there are psychological techniques, like therapy to overcome mood problems and neuroses, or visualisation techniques and positive thinking to improve mental approach.

Meditation

Meditation aims to induce a profound state of both physical and mental relaxation. This state of relaxation is thought to help the body restore its natural healing processes, including those of the immune system. In essence meditation seeks to activate the body's natural 'self-regulating' functions. With repetition, meditation is fairly easy to learn and practice (see page 51), and when practised regularly it can help you to become more relaxed at all times. Studies in the *Journal of Behavioural Medicine* have shown that relaxation can benefit asthma sufferers, and such techniques can help with most symptoms and allergic illnesses.

Creative visualisation

This technique involves using mental imagery to improve your mood and to help symptoms by making positive use of the influence of the mind on the nervous system. The technique has been used to treat both allergic asthma and hay fever. As soon as symptoms begin, the sufferer should clear his or her mind, then start to generate mental images of the different elements of the immune system involved in the allergic reaction, as though directly interacting with and directing them.

For instance, lymphocytes and macrophages could be visualised as dwarfing harmless looking allergens, or the allergens themselves could be imagined transforming from dangerous red to harmless green. Visualisation should be accompanied by constant self-reassurance, and assertions

---

STRESS-BUSTING MASSAGE

Massage is an ideal way to invigorate yourself and relax and tone the muscles of your face and head. The subsequent relaxation and feeling of well-being can help to combat feelings of stress and tiredness by stimulating the circulation of blood to the face and head, leaving you refreshed and alert. Facial massage can also help to relieve headaches that can be brought on by food and environmental allergies.

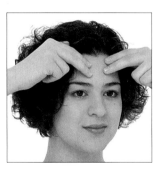

INVIGORATING STIMULATION
Starting with your fingers either side of the bridge of your nose, work in a straight line to the top of your head making small circular movements with your fingers. Continue this all over your scalp.

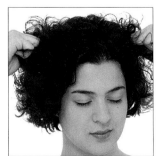

HAIR PULLS
Lay your hands palms down against your scalp and close your hands into fists, gathering up large clumps of hair. Gently but firmly pull your hair until you feel a dragging sensation at the roots. Repeat all over your scalp.

EAR MASSAGE
To complete your facial massage squeeze your ear lobes between fingers and thumbs, rotate the flesh and release. Continue this action around the edge of your ear until you reach the top. Don't pinch your ear or twist it too hard. The acupressure points in the ears relate to every part of the body so you will feel the benefits of ear massage all over.

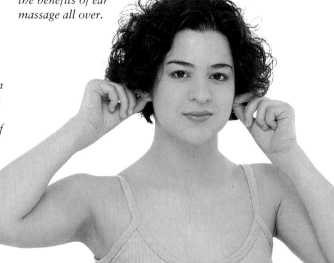

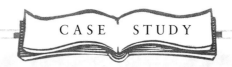
The Hay Fever Sufferer

Hay fever sufferers often find that their conventional drug treatments become increasingly ineffective the more they use them. When this is a problem, sufferers must choose whether to keep increasing the dosage of the drug to maintain its effectiveness or turn to alternative therapies, which offer a more natural approach with relatively few side effects.

Katie is a 25-year-old teacher with a family history of asthma and hay fever. During the past few years she has had regular hay fever starting in May and peaking at the time of her students' exams in late June. She has managed so far with conventional treatment such as antihistamines and steroid nasal sprays, but they have become increasingly less effective. Even the newer antihistamines, which are supposed to be mostly free of side effects, are making her drowsy. Katie fears that this year's heavy load of exam marking will make things almost intolerable. Her GP wants to give her a steroid injection but she is not keen on the idea. A good friend told her about the benefits of homeopathic treatment.

WHAT SHOULD KATIE DO?

First, she should take some basic avoidance measures, such as staying inside when the pollen count is high and changing her clothes when she comes in from outdoors. To take more positive action, she should find a medically qualified homeopathic practitioner who is a registered member of a recognised homeopathic association. In a consultation, the homeopath will listen carefully to Katie's medical history, taking account of details such as the exact timing of her symptoms and her particular physical and emotional reactions at that time. The homeopath will then formulate a prescription and may also suggest ways of dealing with and reducing stress and tension.

Action Plan

LIFESTYLE
Hay fever caused by grass pollens will be mostly confined to the summer, so adopt preventative measures during these months.

STRESS
Adopting a more holistic approach to treatment includes learning to deal with stress and tension, and breaking the vicious cycle that they reinforce.

HEALTH
Rather than resorting to heavy medication, try a more gentle alternative. Properly prepared homeopathic remedies are safe and completely free of side effects.

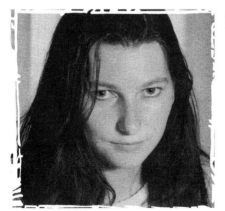

HEALTH
People vary enormously in terms of how they react to medication. Even drugs which should be free of side effects may cause problems for some.

LIFESTYLE
Conventional medicines can be more convenient than other preventative measures but may have side effects. Users can also build up tolerance to drugs, weakening the effects of medication.

STRESS
Allergies can make a stressful situation worse, while increased levels of stress will, in turn, worsen allergies.

HOW THINGS TURNED OUT FOR KATIE

Katie found a homeopath who was also a GP. The homeopath tested Katie for common grass pollens to determine her allergens and prescribed three homeopathic treatments. Her symptoms began to improve within days, and she suffered no side effects. In addition, she learned a deep-breathing technique to help her to relax and deal with stress. When exam marking time came round Katie knew she would be able to cope.

that success is possible. As with other mind therapies, the more often creative visualisation is practised, the easier it will become.

Positive thinking

This technique shares many features with visualisation, but mainly focuses on learning to challenge negative thoughts and to stop attributing negative explanations to events. This means taking a positive view with a positive mental outlook.

For instance, instead of assuming the worst when presented with a potentially allergen-rich environment, view it as a challenge, a chance to assert your control over your allergy. Never focus on past failures, only on your successes and always talk to yourself in a supportive, non-critical way. Negative thinking creates a vicious circle of worsening symptoms and mood. Positive thinking aims to break the cycle, and reverse the trend. Plan allergy treatments and coping strategies for success, and tell yourself that you will achieve your goal. A complete cure is not the aim of this technique, but rather gaining control of your allergy.

HYDROTHERAPY

Two Japanese studies at the Okayama University Medical School in 1992 showed that asthma could be alleviated through spa therapy. Why this should be is not clear, although one suggestion is that the breathing pattern involved in swimming is therapeutic, while the moist, warm air that enters the lungs is soothing. Certainly asthmatics find dry, cold air harsh and irritating. In general, water therapies are relaxing, and exercise is therapeutic for many illnesses.

NATUROPATHY

A naturopath attempts to assess a patient's overall health and well-being, and calls on the full range of alternative therapies to redress any imbalances or problems identified. There is a particular emphasis on nutritional therapy to replace any shortage of nutrients and to cleanse the body of toxins.

Vitamin and mineral deficiencies have been implicated in allergic disease (see page 43), so supplements and nutrient-rich foods are obvious treatments. In particular naturopathy is relevant to the treatment of food allergies and intolerances.

Despite the obvious appeal of this therapy, the wealth of anecdotal support for its efficacy, and a number of clinical studies showing it to be effective, nutritional treatment is still mostly considered to be outside the field of conventional medicine.

ACUPUNCTURE

This ancient Chinese therapy predates recorded Western medicine by at least 2000 years, and is still in regular use in China and around the world today. It is based on the theory that energy or 'chi' flows through the body along energy channels known as meridians. Health problems arise because of the blockages or interruptions in the energy flow. By inserting and manipulating needles at special points this energy can be released and used to heal and relieve discomfort. Traditionally the acupuncturist selects the points requiring treatment on an individual basis. But in the West a more standardised approach is also used, where all patients with the same condition have the same points treated. Both methods seem to work well for pain but the Chinese method seems to be better for allergy treatment.

A number of studies – most of which are Chinese – support the effectiveness of acupuncture. A 1993 trial reported in the *Journal of Traditional Chinese Medicine* showed acupuncture to be superior to IIT in the treatment of acute allergic asthma, rhinitis and chronic urticaria. In Holland about a quarter of general practitioners use acupuncture and believe it to be effective. However, other studies give less impressive results, and cast doubt on the efficacy of acupuncture. On balance it appears that acupuncture can be effective for asthma, and perhaps rhinitis and urticaria, but not all patients benefit.

SPA TREATMENT
This treatment involves swimming and training in a hot pool, while inhaling steam. Studies on the effectiveness of spa treatment back up well-attested anecdotal evidence that swimming is a good exercise for asthmatics (provided they are not allergic to chlorine).

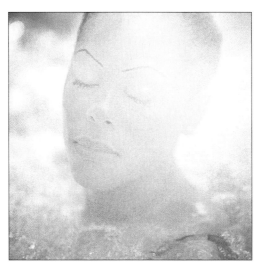

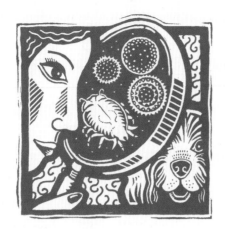

CHAPTER 3

AIRBORNE ALLERGENS

There is a class of allergens which is almost impossible to avoid – the airborne or inhalant allergens. Thousands of tiny particles hang suspended in the air all around us and are taken in with each breath, together with scores of different types of chemical vapours and fumes.

MODERN LIFE AND POLLUTANTS

We live in a complex environment which has changed much during the last century. In particular, the air today is affected by an enormous range of chemicals and biological particles.

Town versus country
Although poor air quality in urban areas is often thought to be the major factor in causing asthma, the changing urban/rural pattern of asthma incidence suggests that industrial and traffic pollution may not be the whole story.

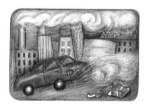

IN TOWN
Asthma does tend to be worse in the polluted air of towns and cities, but the town/country pattern is changing.

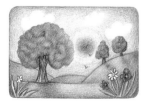

IN THE COUNTRY
There used to be less asthma in rural areas but there are indications that it may be on the increase, for reasons that are not fully understood.

Rising pollution levels and city-wide smog are phenomena which concern everyone. Since the Industrial Revolution of the 19th century, factories, chemical plants, power stations and cars have pumped out smoke and fumes that pose health risks for everyone. Widespread respiratory illness in London in the 1950s (a five-day smog in 1952 killed 4000 people) lead to the Clean Air Act banning the use of domestic coal fires in cities.

At the same time there has been an explosion in the rates of incidence of the commonest forms of allergic reaction – asthma and hay fever (also known as allergic rhinitis). These involve the respiratory system – the mouth, nose, sinuses, throat and lungs – and cause discomfort, disability and even death. Hay fever was unknown until the 19th century, while asthma is becoming a modern plague in developed countries.

These developments have been linked, and doctors and environment campaigners alike call for urgent action to improve air quality and stem the growing tide of respiratory illness. But it seems that outdoor pollution is far from being the whole story. The incidence of asthma is becoming alarmingly high. It is often blamed on traffic fumes but can also be higher in some rural areas than it is in town. On the other hand, hay fever continues to rise in urban areas despite evidence of a fall in the total volume of summer pollens from grasses, trees and flowers in the cities in the past few decades.

Evidence such as this has led experts to look closely at what is happening inside our homes and offices. Just as outdoor pollution has increased over the last hundred years, so modern lifestyles have lead to a radical increase in the levels of indoor pollution.

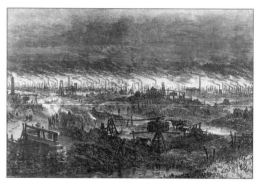

THE BLACK COUNTRY
Industrial pollution was so heavy in this area of the English Midlands that it was nicknamed the Black Country. Breathing problems and lung disease were common local ailments.

INDOOR POLLUTION

Inside our houses there is evidence that there has been an increase in the population of house dust mites within our homes since the 1970s. This decade saw the introduction of heat conservation measures to many houses as a result of the energy crisis.

These measures, such as double glazing and draught proofing, have caused a major increase in the humidity levels in houses, as this humidity is no longer dissipated by the draughts that were characteristic of older, non-insulated houses. Humidity within houses is also increased by boiling water, showers, baths, dishwashers and washing machines, drying clothes and the sweat of humans and pets.

House dust

The house dust mite needs humidity to survive and modern houses and living patterns suit it very well. Large amounts of wall-to-wall carpeting and soft furnishings all encourage the accumulation of house dust and hence the house dust mite. The same conditions also encourage the growth of indoor moulds, another potent source of airborne allergens.

Chemicals

But it seems likely that indoor chemical pollution may be the real culprit behind the modern 'plagues' of respiratory allergies. Attention was drawn to the problem as early as 1962, by the American physician and founder of the clinical ecology (environmental medicine) movement, Dr Theron Randolph. Although he was largely ignored at the time, researchers have by now identified a number of sources of strong indoor chemical pollution.

Natural gas is used for both heating and cooking in a high proportion of homes in the United Kingdom. The fuel is cheap and easy to use, but generates nitrogen dioxide when burnt. Nitrogen dioxide appears to help sensitise a person to other allergens in the atmosphere (see page 62).

The recorded nitrogen dioxide concentrations after a heavy cooking session in kitchens with gas cookers exceed those found in London's Oxford Street on some of the most highly polluted occasions ever recorded there. Because gas is almost odourless, in contrast to vehicle exhaust fumes, this major source of pollution has until recently been overlooked. Calor gas, used in areas where natural gas is not provided by pipeline, produces similar levels of pollution to natural gas. Badly installed or maintained central heating boilers situated in kitchens can also increase pollution.

Perhaps the next most important indoor pollutant is formaldehyde and there has been a huge increase in its use in the past few decades. Formaldehyde was used in cavity wall insulation in the 1970s and 1980s, until it was linked to a series of health problems. After a major scandal in the US, which led to the abandonment of entire housing estates, this use of formaldehyde was stopped. But it is still found in plenty of other places, including fittings and furnishings, carpets, ceiling tiles and cigarette smoke. Carpets can contain a whole cocktail of chemicals, and there are dozens of other chemicals found extensively in houses and offices – in cigarette smoke, household cleaning agents, washing powders, air fresheners, spray perfumes and

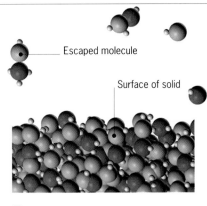

OUTGASSING

Researchers believe that the vapours given off by many synthetic materials, in a process known as outgassing, may be responsible for the development of allergic reactions. Normally the molecules in a solid are bonded together and cannot move very far. But at the surface of any solid, especially synthetic fabrics, soft plastics and glues, a few molecules will escape to exist as vapour.

Escaped molecule

Surface of solid

ESCAPING MOLECULES
In any solid object a few molecules will have enough energy to escape from the surface and exist as gas.

deodorants, paint fumes, floor polishes and in the ink in photocopying machines, for instance. (See page 62 for more details.)

All of these pollutants can now build up inside the home, because the same lack of ventilation that has increased indoor humidity prevents their escape.

ALLERGIES AND MODERN LIVING

So why is this important to allergies? There is evidence that inhalation of chemicals like nitrogen dioxide and formaldehyde (as well as outdoor pollutants like diesel particles) can affect the immune system so that it is more likely to produce an allergic reaction to normally harmless substances, like house dust or mould spores, which it should ignore. The immune systems of infants are less able to recognise which substances are harmless and which are dangerous, and so young children may be particularly vulnerable to this kind of interference. If further research confirms this theory, it is possible that air pollution, particularly indoor air pollution, should be considered as one of the major health threats in the developed world. The chemicals to which we are unwittingly exposed could be sensitising us to the increasingly high levels of biological and chemical particles in the air – both outside and inside our homes.

PAINT HAZARD
Common household substances like paint can give off fumes composed of a cocktail of synthetic chemicals. These continue to be given off even after the paint has dried.

COMMON INHALANT ALLERGENS

Probably the best-known allergy is hay fever, usually caused by pollen. But pollen is just one of a host of airborne allergens that can cause nasal symptoms and other allergic reactions.

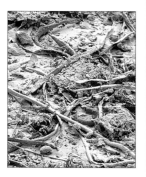

HOUSE DUST
Household dust is a complex mixture of many things, such as grit, skin cells from humans and pets, mould spores and fragments of insects.

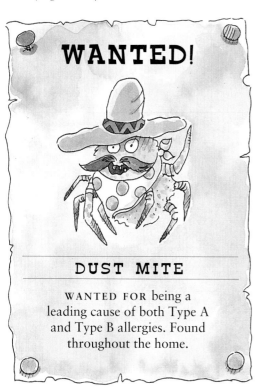

WANTED!

DUST MITE

WANTED FOR being a leading cause of both Type A and Type B allergies. Found throughout the home.

The respiratory system includes the inside of the nose, the sinuses, throat and lungs. These surfaces all come into contact with the air that we breathe, and thus with the enormous range of chemicals, vapours and particles that are found in the atmosphere.

DUST AND THE HOUSE DUST MITE

The melange of ingredients that makes up house dust is one of the leading causes of nasal problems (known as rhinitis) and asthma. Amongst many other things, dust contains house dust mite droppings which can produce an allergic response. Sufferers are affected to some extent throughout the year. In the UK the commonest dust mite is *Dermatophagoides pteronnyssinus*; in the US the most common type of dust mite is *Dermatophagoides farinae*. The word 'dermatophagoides' means 'skin eater' and this microscopic organism feeds off discarded skin flakes, which we constantly shed. There are more than two million house dust mites in the average double mattress and it has been calculated that 10 per cent of the weight of an average pillow consists of house dust mites and the dead skin cells that they feed on. Each dust mite produces about twenty faecal pellets every day.

Ideal home

Mattresses and pillows are the soft furnishings with which human beings have the most constant and intimate contact. We spend an average of eight hours a day in bed and while in bed we are warm and frequently sweaty. Humidity is vital for the health and survival of dust mites, so pillows, moistened by damp breath and sweat throughout the night, are the ideal place for them to flourish. This is one reason why asthma is often worse at night. Other habitats which suit mites are soft carpets and any soft and upholstered furnishings.

Mites will flourish more in houses with poor ventilation and high humidity – also conditions that encourage the growth of moulds. Both can be largely eliminated if the ventilation is good enough.

MOULDS

Very few people are aware of the presence of moulds in the air that they breathe, but numerically there are about fifty times more mould spores in the atmosphere than there is grass pollen at the height of the season. Moulds need warmth and humidity to survive and outdoor moulds are most prevalent in the summer and the autumn. There is a major decrease in the mould count with the onset of the first frost of winter.

DID YOU KNOW?

Although each house dust mite is only 0.2 mm long, it has been estimated that if all the mites in an average double bed were laid out nose to tail, they would stretch the length of five football pitches.

Indoor moulds are as much of a problem as outdoor ones, and in damp houses problems with moulds can exist throughout the year, especially with the mould Penicillium, which is the one responsible for the green, furry growths on stale bread.

Outdoor moulds are more difficult to avoid than house dust and house dust mites, but there are steps you can take to limit the provocation of your symptoms by moulds (see pages 64–67).

POLLEN

It is usually fairly obvious when pollen allergy is a part or the whole cause of the problem. Symptoms related solely to pollen sensitivity will be restricted entirely to the 'season' of that pollen, and in the United Kingdom, for example, the pollen seasons are fairly well delineated. Allergists often use 'pollen calendars' to help them diagnose a patient's particular trigger. Once they have done this they may offer desensitisation to help pollen sufferers (see Chapter 2).

The most common pollen allergens are the grasses, which cause clinical hay fever, but some cases of asthma are also limited to these months of the year. Pollen can also cause other symptoms, for instance chronic fatigue states which only occur in these specific months and can be provoked by skin tests with certain summer pollen.

ASTHMA ATTACK!

Following a thunderstorm in London in June 1994 over 600 people filled emergency rooms suffering from asthma. Reports in the March 1996 issue of the *British Medical Journal* suggested that the cause was a combination of high pollen count and the weather conditions of the storm. High moisture levels could have caused pollen to rupture, releasing smaller particles which can be inhaled more deeply, causing worse reactions.

Season of illness

An idea about which specific type of pollen is involved can be reached by carefully recording the months in which the symptoms occur. This is reasonably easy when, for example, the asthma or rhinitis is entirely related to the summer months, but it is much more difficult if year-round allergens are operating at the same time.

As a general rule, if a patient has symptoms limited to March, April and May, the culprits are usually tree pollen. The most common trees involved are birch, beech, alder, oak, hazel, ash, plane and poplar. These trees are all wind pollinated and the pollen is widely distributed. It is said that

MOULD ALLERGY WARNING SIGNS

Apart from skin testing, there are a number of observable signs that a person is mould sensitive. In particular, symptoms tend to be worse in damp homes or certain outdoor situations:

▶ *In warm, humid or rainy conditions and especially if the sufferer is near deciduous trees.*

▶ *Just before a thunderstorm, when the rise in humidity induces moulds to release their spores.*

▶ *Anywhere near harvesting, but especially near combine harvesters, which throw up huge clouds of mould spores.*

▶ *When compost heaps are turned over – this releases a huge cloud of mould spores.*

▶ *When leaves are raked – rotting leaves are covered with moulds.*

POLLEN AND THE SEASONS

Flowering plants – which includes most deciduous trees – use pollen to spread their male gametes (the plant equivalent of sperm). Different plants release pollen at different times of the year, and many hay fever sufferers find that their symptoms are worse in, or are entirely restricted to, a few months of the year – the months when their trigger plant is in season. When this is depends on where you are: northerly countries have shorter springs and summers, while tropical countries have extended growing seasons.

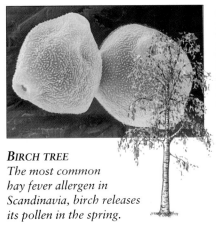

BIRCH TREE
The most common hay fever allergen in Scandinavia, birch releases its pollen in the spring.

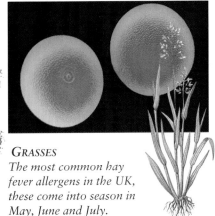

GRASSES
The most common hay fever allergens in the UK, these come into season in May, June and July.

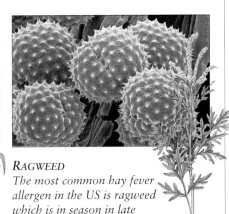

RAGWEED
The most common hay fever allergen in the US is ragweed which is in season in late summer.

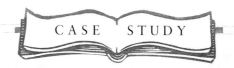

The Wheezy Child

Many allergy sufferers have to deal with more than one allergic condition, and the cumulative effects can be very painful and distressing. Children, in particular, can suffer physically, emotionally and socially. Being excluded from normal childhood activities can create stress which serves to worsen allergic conditions.

Olivia is seven years old and suffers from both asthma and hay fever. Her family have recently moved house. Building work in their new home has thrown up a lot of dust, and there are high levels of chemicals and vapours in the air, derived from fresh paint and varnish, and outgassing from new furniture. Olivia has also changed schools, and feels nervous about her new surroundings and classmates. She is keen to join in with games but her asthma prevents this and she feels left out as a result. The family doctor has prescribed conventional medication, but it hasn't eased Olivia's distress at the frequency of her attacks. The GP has suggested consulting a naturopath to investigate preventative measures.

WHAT SHOULD OLIVIA DO?

The naturopath identified Olivia's home environment as her major source of problems, and suggested that her bedroom be made into a dust and fume-free zone. The naturopath also recognised that when Olivia was tense or nervous she was less able to cope with her attacks and they also lasted much longer. He discovered that her diet was rather low in zinc and magnesium, both of which help to regulate the immune system response. The naturopath recommended some dietary changes to Olivia's mother, including wheatgerm and sunflower seeds for zinc and bananas for magnesium. Together the three of them practised breathing and relaxation techniques.

Action Plan

DIET
Increase intake of zinc and magnesium to regulate and boost immune system.

STRESS
Practise breathing exercises to help calm the body and exert more control over the respiratory system.

HOME
Make the bedroom a dust-free, fume-free environment, and improve ventilation in the rest of the house. Restrict use of paint, varnish and other chemicals which may give off fumes and vapours.

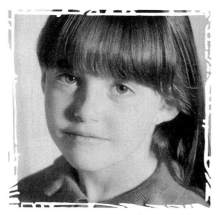

DIET
Deficiencies in essential nutrients can increase the frequency of allergic attacks as well as their severity.

STRESS
Tension and fear can heighten respiratory problems as the body hyperventilates in response to stress.

HOME
Dust and chemical fumes can seriously exacerbate asthma attacks and other allergic conditions.

HOW THINGS TURNED OUT FOR OLIVIA

Improved ventilation and a vacuum fitted with a filter helped to clear dust, fumes and vapours from Olivia's home. Over the next few months Olivia's mother noticed a decrease in the severity and frequency of her asthma attacks. Her diet has improved, with a higher zinc and magnesium intake, and the breathing exercises help Olivia to cope with feelings of panic during an attack. Now she can take part in games.

some tree pollen can travel up to 160 km (100 miles). Most allergy clinics stock individual extracts of the major wind-pollinating trees, so that the individual's specific sensitivities can be discovered through skin tests (see Chapter 2). In contrast, other trees are insect pollinated. Cherry is a good example of an insect-pollinated tree and its pollen rarely gives people problems unless they are literally standing under the tree.

Symptoms which occur predominantly in June and July are nearly always caused by grass pollen, although some early sporing moulds can cause some confusion in this respect. A small number of sufferers have problems limited to August and September and these are usually caused by reactions to nettles, mugwort, plantains or dock pollen, or ragweed in North America. Flowers are seasonal, but most are insect-pollinated, which means that their pollen is not designed to be dispersed by wind, so they are not usually a problem.

ANIMALS

Allergies can be caused by a whole range of animals, including cats, dogs, horses, hamsters, gerbils, guinea pigs, rats and mice. The urine of small creatures like hamsters and mice is a common allergic trigger. However, cat allergen is the most pervasive and persistent and the commonest cause of problems for sufferers of asthma and rhinitis – in some sufferers even the smallest amount of allergen carried on the clothes of a pet owner is enough to set off an attack.

Cats

After a cat licks itself microscopic specks of dried saliva are given off to the atmosphere. These contain a protein which is the main allergen for those affected by cats. As the particles are very small and light they can stay airborne for many hours and the protein spreads itself everywhere, coating the walls, windows and furniture. Cat salivary protein can still be detected several years after a cat has vacated a house, so even if a cat is got rid of in an attempt to cure an allergy the house will need to be thoroughly cleaned. This means washing all curtains and fabrics, shampooing the carpets and washing the walls. In particular cats should not be allowed into a sufferer's bedroom.

Dogs

In general, dogs are less of a problem for allergy sufferers than cats. Dog allergens are present in their skin particles and saliva. These allergenic particles become attached to fur, which therefore carries the allergen but is not allergenic in itself. If the problem is bad enough some hard decisions might have to be taken and the dog may have to go. As with cats, however, desensitisation or the use of measures to limit the effect of the animals on the allergy sufferer may work well enough to enable the pet to stay.

CHEMICALS AND GASES

There are many chemicals that seem to be involved in producing allergic reactions. The precise role of each one is unclear.

CAT-ASTROPHE!

Cats clean themselves by licking, which means that their fur is covered in saliva. When this dries and flakes off it can get anywhere in the house – even on the walls. The cat basket, furniture that gets rubbed against, and any of your pet's favourite napping spots are all danger areas for cat allergens.

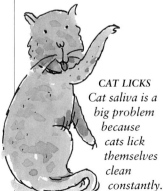

CAT LICKS
Cat saliva is a big problem because cats lick themselves clean constantly.

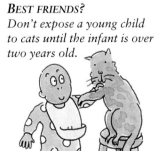

BEST FRIENDS?
Don't expose a young child to cats until the infant is over two years old.

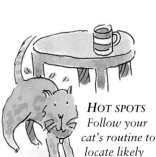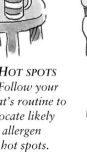

HOT SPOTS
Follow your cat's routine to locate likely allergen hot spots.

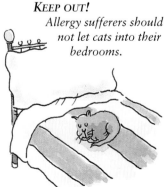

KEEP OUT!
Allergy sufferers should not let cats into their bedrooms.

GAS COOKERS

While gas boilers are likely to be vented to the outside, gas hobs release their fumes directly into the air. Extractor fans, or an extractor hood, vented to the outside, can help reduce nitrogen dioxide levels in the kitchen.

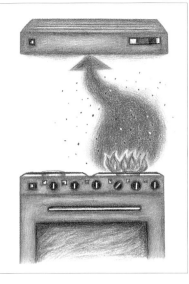

VAPOURS AND FUMES
Natural gas burns to give large quantities of nitrogen dioxide, together with other oxides of nitrogen, which may have similar allergy-triggering effects.

Toxic molecules

Paint is usually made from organic compounds derived from crude oil. It often contains potentially allergenic, toxic or irritant chemicals like toluene.

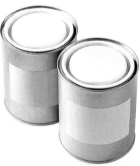

PAINT
Substances like toluene, which is used as a solvent, can outgas into the atmosphere.

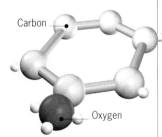

Carbon

Oxygen

TOLUENE MOLECULE
When toluene outgasses it can cause problems for allergy sufferers.

Some may cause allergies directly by acting as allergens. Others have toxic or pseudo-allergic effects. Some may lead to the development of allergies because of the way in which they interfere with the immune system and result in an inappropriate defensive reaction to protect the body (see page 57).

Nitrogen dioxide

High on the list of chemicals that can interfere with the immune system is nitrogen dioxide. This gas is present in car exhaust fumes and is also produced in large quantities by gas cookers. If an individual inhales nitrogen dioxide it can irritate the nose and the adjacent upper respiratory system. If an antigen like house dust mite is then inhaled the individual may become sensitised and allergic to it, which might not have happened in the normal course of events. (It should be noted that this effect has only been observed in research involving mice and rats. Whether the same effect occurs in human beings is not yet known.)

Studies reported in *The Lancet* show that normal domestic levels of nitrogen dioxide enhance the adverse response to inhaled house dust mite in patients with mild asthma. A recent study of 15 000 adults, published in *The Lancet* in February 1996, showed evidence of an association between the incidence and severity of asthma in young adults and the use of gas cookers.

Other gases

A 1995 Swedish study found significant relationships between nocturnal breathlessness and indoor concentrations of carbon dioxide, formaldehyde and volatile organic compounds (VOCs) such as phenol and ethanol. The study concluded that VOCs and formaldehyde were likely to cause asthmatic symptoms and that there was a need to increase ventilation and reduce wall-to-wall carpeting and dampness.

Sulphur dioxide is another gas linked with damage to the immune system making the development of allergies more likely. It was a major industrial pollutant earlier this century, and is also a product of car exhausts.

Other chemicals

Other chemicals particularly associated with allergy problems include trichlorethylene which is used in carpet shampoo, dry cleaning fluids, floor polish, photocopying machines, furniture glues, and various machine oils and oil solvents.

Phenol is one of the chemicals given off when plastics 'outgas', or release molecules into the air as vapour (see page 57). The softer the plastic and the greater the heat, the faster the plastic outgasses. Department stores, where there are many soft plastic coverings, have a lot of this vapour, especially when it is very warm. Phenol derives from benzene, itself a carcinogenic (cancer-causing) substance, and is toxic.

Xylene is a chemical derived from benzene, which outgasses from products such as paint, especially gloss paint. Patients who notice symptoms like headaches, fatigue or wheezing when gloss paint is first applied are usually reacting to another benzene-derivative component called toluene.

Studies on mice have shown that fine particles from the exhausts of diesel engines are capable of interfering with the response of the immune system, enhancing its tendency to be hypersensitive, perhaps through a similar mechanism to the effects of indoor nitrogen dioxide pollution.

CIGARETTE SMOKE

Numerous studies of the links between asthma and cigarette smoke show that smoking, either active or passive, is a major cause of asthma and other symptoms of allergy. Cigarette smoke is a potent mixture of some 3600 complex chemicals, including at least 43 known carcinogens (including tar, benzene and nitrosamines). Asthmatics who inhale cigarette fumes, actively or passively, put themselves at risk.

ASTHMA AND COMMON VAPOURS

In a study carried out in New York at the Albert Einstein School of Medicine and published in the *American Journal of Medicine*, asthmatic patients were exposed to a range of common odours under controlled conditions. The results were remarkably consistent. Of the 60 asthmatic patients surveyed, 57 complained of respiratory reactions on exposure to common odours. For example, exposure to a small amount of atomised cologne caused an 18 to 58 per cent drop in the breathing capacity of susceptible subjects, and made them complain of chest tightening and wheezing within 1 to 2 minutes of exposure.

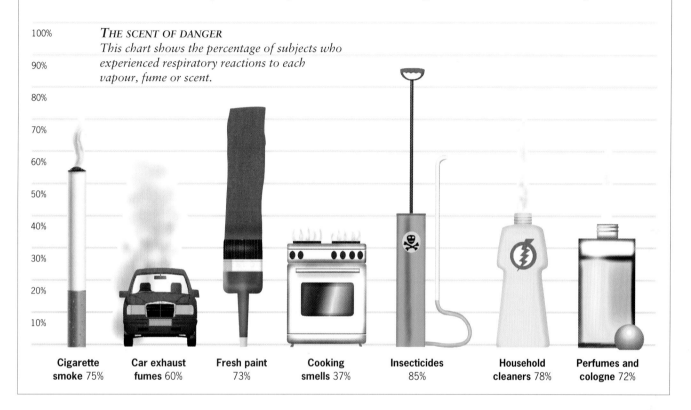

THE SCENT OF DANGER
This chart shows the percentage of subjects who experienced respiratory reactions to each vapour, fume or scent.

Cigarette smoke 75%	**Car exhaust fumes** 60%	**Fresh paint** 73%	**Cooking smells** 37%	**Insecticides** 85%	**Household cleaners** 78%	**Perfumes and cologne** 72%

ASTHMA AND POLLUTION

More than 12 per cent of children in the UK now have asthma, and it is also on the increase in adults – between 1500 and 2000 people die from asthma every year in the UK alone. Outdoor pollutants – in particular diesel and petrol fumes, ozone and sulphur dioxide emissions – can precipitate asthma in sensitive subjects. Evidence that asthma was increasing while overall air pollution was dropping has led some researchers to play down the role of outdoor pollution.

For instance, the apparently unpolluted Isle of Skye has a higher rate of asthma than that of many industrial cities like Aberdeen and Cardiff. In practice, though, the cases of asthma on Skye are concentrated around the port area, which has a high level of diesel pollution. Diesel fumes contain millions of diesel particulates – tiny particles which can get deep into the lungs and are very harmful. There are an increasing number of diesel vehicles around, and similar particles are emitted from some power stations. In other words, outdoor pollution can play a major role in causing asthma.

But indoor pollutants are often more important. Cigarette smoke, moulds, mites and volatile vapours from perfumes, toiletries and cleaning and DIY products can all provoke asthma. This source of pollution can be reduced by simple changes such as increasing ventilation and choosing products with no chemical smell.

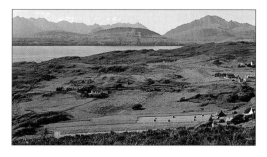

THE ISLE OF SKYE
Skye is famed for its unspoilt scenery but the high rate of asthma there was a puzzle until it was found that most cases were concentrated around the port, with its diesel vessels.

PREVENTATIVE MEASURES

Preventative measures to reduce levels of airborne allergens, and your exposure to them, are the key to managing and reducing the symptoms of inhalant allergy.

The first step towards finding effective preventative measures is to identify your trigger or triggers so that you know what you have to avoid. The history and pattern of your symptoms should indicate whether your allergy is caused by an inhalant, but it may require an expert to pin down exactly what you are allergic to. Allergists and some GPs stock a range of extracts for carrying out skin tests, or they may use a RAST test to confirm their diagnosis (although negative results cannot rule out an allergic reaction). Or you could try an alternative practitioner, although the reliability of their tests will not have been confirmed by recognised clinical methods (see Chapter 2).

UNIVERSAL MEASURES

Some of the preventative measures you can take apply equally well to most indoor inhalant allergens. Moulds and mites both thrive in the same conditions, and measures to clean up the air in your home generally to create a hypo-allergenic environment will combat excess humidity, chemical vapours and particles (see pages 66–67).

Reducing dampness

Damp conditions favour both moulds and mites, so reducing humidity levels in the home can really help allergy sufferers. Firstly, cut down on the amount of moisture that gets into the house to start with; secondly, reduce moisture and condensation within the house; and thirdly, increase ventilation so that moisture can escape. Reducing dampness can involve making some major alterations, but simple tactics can also make a difference.

Controlling dust mites

An international workshop in 1988 suggested that a tenfold reduction in mite allergen exposure was required to improve symptoms. Steps you can take to achieve this involve changing your home environment so that it does not favour dust mites, and attacking the mites directly to kill them and remove their allergenic debris.

Eliminating mould

Mould spores can make a significant contribution to an allergy sufferer's allergen load (the total amount of triggers a sufferer's immune system has to deal with) if moulds are allowed to flourish in the home. Reduce overall levels of moisture and eliminate likely sites of mould growth, such as old food or pot plants.

MATTRESS AND PILLOW COVERS

After increasing ventilation in your house, the single most important measure you can take against house dust mites is to enclose both mattress and pillows in microporous covers. These are made from material which has holes (pores) small enough to prevent dust mites or their droppings from getting in or out, but big enough to let water vapour through. The covers fit onto mattresses, pillows and duvets; sheets, pillow cases and duvet covers go on top.

DID YOU KNOW?
There are more mould spores in the air than any other biological particle. The record mould spore count in the British Isles is 160 000 per m³ of air. The record pollen count is just 2800 per m³.

HYPO-ALLERGENIC BEDDING
Pillows and duvets stuffed with hypo-allergenic filler material can be encased in mite-proof cases and covers which seal out dust mites, but do not trap moisture.

Better than plastic

Previously, plastic mattress covers were used as anti-mite measures. They were completely impermeable, however, and a drop in temperature would produce condensation on the inside of the cover. This in turn could lead to the growth of moulds, which could then become a major problem if any small holes developed in the cover.

Ideally you should invest in a new mattress when you get the covers. If you are using an existing mattress you should vacuum it thoroughly before putting on the cover. Make sure you wash your bedding frequently to prevent dust-mite-attracting skin cells from building up.

DAMP DUSTING

Dusting with a feather duster simply puts more dust and mould spores into the air. To remove dust effectively you need to use a damp cloth; rinse it under a tap and don't dry it inside the house. Better still, use a high quality vacuum cleaner to get rid of dust.

DEHUMIDIFIERS

These machines are very useful for reducing humidity, thus making the environment less attractive to dust mites and mould. All dehumidifiers use the same technology as refrigerators and work by cooling air. As the air cools, water condenses out of it and is collected in a tank.

Relatively low-powered dehumidifiers are sold widely in high street stores, but specialist firms supplying machines for allergy sufferers sell much more powerful models. Air conditioners have much the same effect, but are more expensive.

MITE KILLING TREATMENTS

A study published in the journal *Clinical and Experimental Allergy* in 1995 showed that steam cleaning was very effective at killing mites in carpets. Alternative treatments include chemicals that kill mites – known as acaricides – but these can cause reactions, and studies have shown them to give disappointing results.

Liquid nitrogen

Liquid nitrogen is a very effective anti-mite treatment – it is extremely cold and freezes the dust mites to death. Liquid nitrogen does not damage carpets or upholstery, but can be very dangerous, and has to be

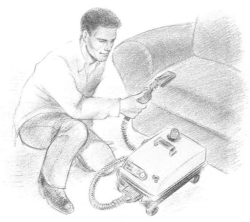

MITE BLASTER
Steam cleaners use superheated steam to kill dust mites. You can buy or hire steam cleaners from specialist suppliers.

handled by trained personnel. The treatment needs to be repeated roughly every six months and must be followed by very careful vacuuming.

HYPO-ALLERGENIC VACUUM CLEANERS

Standard vacuum cleaners are not much use for reducing levels of dust and dust mites. The collecting bags have small pores which allow microscopic dust mite droppings to escape. These are then expelled from the vacuum cleaner via the exhaust and often increase the amount of allergen suspended in the air. Many patients who are allergic to mites report illness after vacuum cleaning.

There is now a range of vacuum cleaners designed to eliminate this effect. Some use very high quality bags, which retain the allergenic particles and are backed up by a high quality filter (a HEPA filter) that cleans the exhaust air before it leaves the machine. Others pass the exhaust through water. A cheaper, but less effective, compromise is to buy a filter and fit it to your existing vacuum cleaner.

AIR FILTERS

There are three main types of machine that are used to clean air: ionisers, electrostatic air cleaners and HEPA filter air cleaners. Air filters tend to be noisy, so it is worth trying one on approval before buying. Improving ventilation in the home, particularly the bedroom, may eliminate the need for a filter. However, if you also want to reduce chemical pollution, the air filter

LOW EMISSION VACUUM CLEANERS
Normal vacuums allow tiny particles to slip through the bag, which remain suspended in the air for up to 8 hours. Allergy sufferers can benefit from a cleaner which captures and retains these particles.

Hypo-allergenic Home

Keeping your home free of allergens is a difficult task, but there are dozens of ways you can fight dust mites and moulds, improve ventilation, keep out dampness and cope with pets.

The first line of battle in the war against allergens is at home. Modern housing tends to restrict the circulation of air, and may even be geared specifically to prevent air (and therefore heat) from getting in or out. This helps moulds and dust mites by preventing the escape of moisture, and also leads to the build-up of fumes and vapours. People with severe, chronic allergic symptoms may be prepared to go to any lengths to improve conditions in their home, but most of the steps outlined here do not involve major modifications. Follow the checklists to make sure that you are not missing any out.

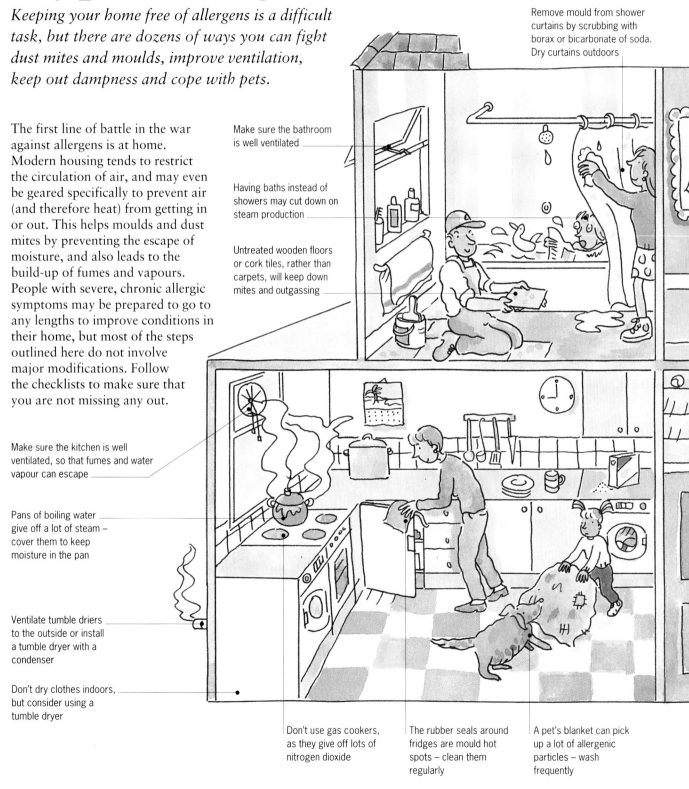

Remove mould from shower curtains by scrubbing with borax or bicarbonate of soda. Dry curtains outdoors

Make sure the bathroom is well ventilated

Having baths instead of showers may cut down on steam production

Untreated wooden floors or cork tiles, rather than carpets, will keep down mites and outgassing

Make sure the kitchen is well ventilated, so that fumes and water vapour can escape

Pans of boiling water give off a lot of steam – cover them to keep moisture in the pan

Ventilate tumble driers to the outside or install a tumble dryer with a condenser

Don't dry clothes indoors, but consider using a tumble dryer

Don't use gas cookers, as they give off lots of nitrogen dioxide

The rubber seals around fridges are mould hot spots – clean them regularly

A pet's blanket can pick up a lot of allergenic particles – wash frequently

Pot plants are a potent source of mould growth. Put a thick layer of sand on the soil, and water from the bottom.

Open the windows to let out fumes and dampness (but hay fever sufferers should keep them closed in pollen season)

Use mite-proof coverings for mattress, duvet and pillows

Keep pets out of bedrooms

Electric blankets reduce mattress humidity, lowering levels of mites

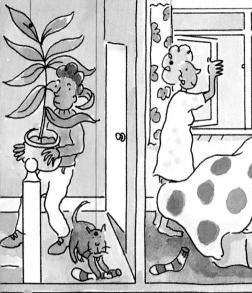
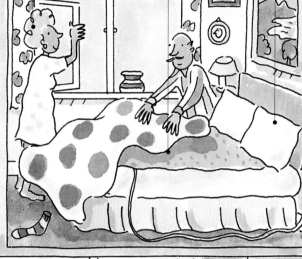
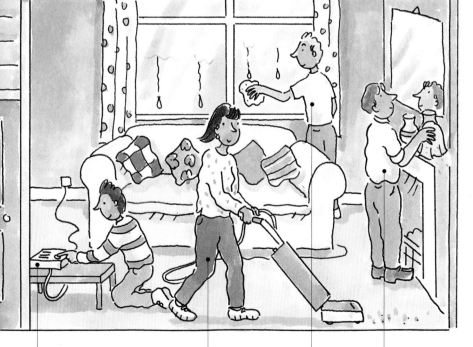

Purify the air with a combined HEPA and activated carbon air filter

Vacuum frequently with a cleaner which has a HEPA filter fitted

Mop up any condensation that occurs on window sills and remove any mould

When dusting use a damp cloth, rinse it under the tap and dry it outside

REDUCING DAMPNESS

▶ *Check that the fabric of the house is sound, especially the roof and the guttering.*

▶ *To prevent rising damp and water penetrating through walls consider a chemical damp course – silicone compounds, either sprayed onto walls or injected into them. The compounds harden into a waterproof layer.*

▶ *Damp spots can be treated by exposure to light and dry heat, and anti-mould measures.*

▶ *Use dehumidifiers (see page 65).*

▶ *Install trickle vents around the windows to let moist air out continually.*

CONTROLLING DUST MITES

▶ *Increase ventilation.*

▶ *Hot washing (higher than 58°C/135°F) will kill mites.*

▶ *Steam cleaning is highly effective for killing mites. Liquid nitrogen treatment is a specialist alternative. Tannic acid treats mite droppings.*

ELIMINATING MOULD

▶ *Make sure no food is allowed to go mouldy within the house.*

▶ *Use mould retarding sprays or solutions such as borax (available from hardware stores) for the bottom of windows, between bathroom tiles and on baths.*

CUT DOWN ON CHEMICALS

▶ *Don't use fabric conditioners or enzymatic washing powders. Avoid strong-smelling cleaning products.*

▶ *Don't use air fresheners or perfumes.*

▶ *Avoid particle boards and synthetic materials.*

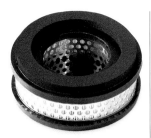

***HEPA** FILTERS*
High Efficiency Particle Air filters are made of glass fibres less than one micron thick, embedded in a matrix made from larger fibres.

should have an activated carbon filter. Ionisers and electrostatic filters have flaws which limit their usefulness to allergy sufferers. Ionisers are cheap but generally too small to make much improvement in air quality. There has been no convincing medical proof demonstrating that ionisers help people suffering from asthma. In fact, the ionisation process can produce ozone which itself can trigger an asthma attack. Electrostatic air cleaners are effective for removing smoke and are popular in pubs and restaurants. However, they require regular cleaning and have a very limited effect on airborne bacteria, viruses and odours.

HEPA air filters

HEPA air filters force air through a filter which physically traps airborne pollutants. The greater the surface area of the HEPA filter, the better that filter will perform. It has been shown that the best quality (but therefore most expensive) HEPA filters are more beneficial to asthma and other allergy sufferers than other types of air filter.

To clear chemical pollution from the air you also need a good activated carbon filter, which is usually combined with a HEPA filter – available from specialist suppliers.

TANNIC ACID TREATMENT

Tannic acid is a widely available and relatively cheap treatment which makes mite droppings less allergenic, rather than actually killing mites. It is sprayed onto carpets and upholstery, dries to a fine powder and is then vacuumed off. One treatment can be effective for up to three months.

REDUCING INDOOR CHEMICAL POLLUTION

Chemical pollution comes from materials used in building, furnishings, varnishes and paint, from products used for cleaning, freshening and so on, and from the gas or oil used for heating and cooking.

Domestic gas and oil

Gas cookers give off high levels of noxious fumes (see page 62). If these cause you problems the most effective answer is to switch to electricity. Gas boilers and heaters which are well-installed and maintained, and are vented to the outside, cause problems less frequently. If they do you could consider having the central heating boiler moved to an outhouse or properly ventilated boiler room, or install electric heating. Remove gas fires, if possible, or take steps to improve the ventilation of the room.

Before embarking on any major alterations, however, make sure that it really is gas that is causing the problem. Turn off your gas supply for at least ten days and evaluate your response. The same considerations apply with oil heaters. Obviously this may be very inconvenient and will require some forward planning, such as waiting for warm weather and getting hold of some alternative electric appliances.

Formaldehyde

Formaldehyde can be hard to deal with since it may be present in furnishings and carpets. Before getting rid of furnishings, evaluate your response to their absence by putting them in a garage or someone else's house for at least two weeks. If you have to replace carpet then consider getting rid of wall-to-wall carpets altogether, as this will help with mites as well. Real wood, ceramic and cork tiles should be free from formaldehyde (but remember that many varnishes can cause problems). Use rugs that you can wash frequently.

DEALING WITH PETS

The hair and dander – flakes of dried skin – shed by pets can be a particular problem for allergy sufferers. Exclude any pet from the bedroom, day and night, clean its blanket weekly and improve ventilation in the house. Desensitisation treatment may help.

WELL GROOMED
Use a hand held vacuum cleaner, or a special attachment, to vacuum dander and hair directly from your pet, if possible. Get someone who isn't allergic to give your pet a good grooming – out of doors!

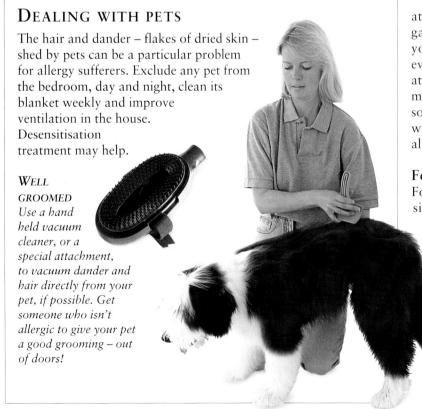

HAY FEVER AND PERENNIAL RHINITIS

Allergic rhinitis is one of the most common allergic complaints, causing discomfort and misery to millions. When symptoms are seasonal and pollen is to blame, rhinitis is called hay fever.

Allergic rhinitis is the inflammation of the mucous membranes lining the nose and sinuses (see below). The inflammation can be caused by a variety of inhaled vapours and particles. These act as irritants or allergens, triggering the mast cells in the nasal lining to release their cargo of histamine. Inflammation and excessive secretion of mucus result.

Hay fever was effectively unknown until the early 19th century, when London doctor John Bostock described his own symptoms. At first the disease was known as Bostock's catarrh, but the public linked the increasingly common condition with the 'effluvium from new hay', and the press coined the term 'hay fever'. In practice, fever is a comparatively rare symptom – it is the respiratory tract which is most affected.

SYMPTOMS

Typically, symptoms include sneezing and runny or blocked nasal passages. The eyes may be affected, and may run or itch. The palate of the mouth is frequently itchy as well. Surrounding parts of the upper respiratory tract like the sinuses and the Eustachian tubes can become involved, causing painful sinuses or impaired hearing.

Triggers of rhinitis

Rhinitis can be divided into 'perennial rhinitis', where the symptoms persist throughout the year, and 'seasonal rhinitis' (often more severe), where the symptoms are limited to the summer months. The latter is what people mean when they say 'hay fever'.

Seasonal rhinitis is usually caused by pollen from plants which come into season in summer and early spring, or sometimes by spores from seasonal moulds, more likely during autumn months. Different types of plants release their pollen in different months (see page 59), so the months when symptoms are worst can give clues as to what sort of plant is responsible.

Mould spores and pollen are by no means the only triggers of rhinitis. House dust mites, pet allergens and all the other airborne allergens can be responsible, particularly for perennial rhinitis because they are in the environment all year round.

Food triggers

Any foods can trigger rhinitis, just as they can asthma. Some foods may also cause cross-reactions in which people who are allergic to a particular plant's pollen may react to foods made from related plants. For instance, someone allergic to mugwort pollen may also react to camomile tea, made

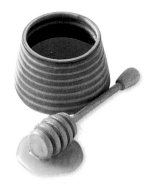

CROSS-REACTIVE
Allergies can be complex, and surprising links can sometimes be found between airborne allergens and food allergens. For instance, ragwort pollen can cross-react with honey.

AFFECTED AREAS IN RHINITIS

Rhinitis causes inflammation of the mucous membranes that line the nose and the sinuses – air-filled cavities within the skull which keep it lightweight, and provide space for the human voice to resonate. Inflammation causes itchiness and excessive mucus production.

Blocked frontal sinus

Blocked sphenoidal sinus

Blocked maxillary sinus

Watery eyes

Blocked ethmoidal sinus

Blocked Eustachian tube

Irritated throat

RELATED PARTS
Other affected areas include the throat, Eustachian tubes and eyes.

Strategies for
Avoiding Pollen

For most people summer is a time to enjoy being outdoors, but for hay fever sufferers it can be a season of misery. However, there are some strategies you can follow to reduce pollen levels in your immediate environment.

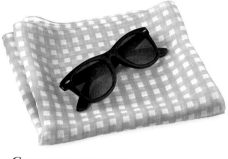

GLASSES AND SCARVES
If you do have to go outside, some simple precautions can help to keep pollen away from your nose, mouth and eyes. Wear sunglasses to protect your eyes (special sunglasses are available from specialist suppliers), and a mask across your nose and mouth – a scarf makes a more stylish accessory. A scarf worn on the head will help to keep pollen out of your hair.

HOW DOES YOUR GARDEN GROW?
By minimising local sources of pollen – your garden – and keeping pollen out of the house, you can make an allergen-free oasis for yourself.

There is not much you can do about the levels of pollen in the atmosphere outside your home, car or office, but there are a number of steps you can take to minimise the amount of allergen that invades your living and working space. Air filters and conditioners can help to clear the air in your home, office and particularly your car. When you go inside you carry a cargo of pollen stuck to your hair and clothes. Rinsing or washing these can help to keep the pollen out. Mow the lawn frequently. Consider converting your garden into an allergen-free one by replacing lawn with a rock garden or patio. This will also reduce the need for pesticides and other chemicals. When you have to go outside, avoid walking past fields and grassy areas, keep an eye on the pollen forecasts and learn the conditions that spell danger: dry, windy days, and early mornings and late evenings. Plan journeys accordingly.

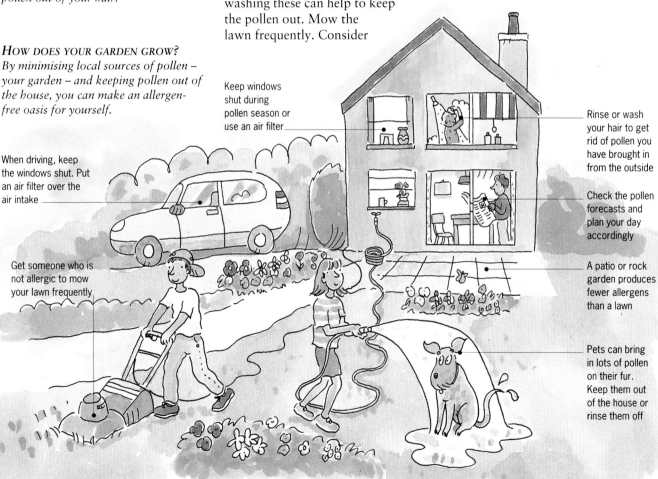

Keep windows shut during pollen season or use an air filter

When driving, keep the windows shut. Put an air filter over the air intake

Get someone who is not allergic to mow your lawn frequently

Rinse or wash your hair to get rid of pollen you have brought in from the outside

Check the pollen forecasts and plan your day accordingly

A patio or rock garden produces fewer allergens than a lawn

Pets can bring in lots of pollen on their fur. Keep them out of the house or rinse them off

70

from a plant in the same family. In some cases there is no relation between the different families – for instance, birch pollen sensitivity is linked to food allergy to walnut, apple, carrot, cherry, and many others.

DRUG-FREE REMEDIES

Conventional medication for hay fever and rhinitis has side effects which can create almost as much discomfort as the allergy itself. But there are other ways to relieve the irritating symptoms of rhinitis.

The usual prescription for hay fever is antihistamine which effectively relieves symptoms but tends to cause drowsiness and dry out the mucous membranes. The mucus also becomes thick and clogs up the sinus or respiratory tract, resulting in a dry cough. Nasal decongestants can clear up sinusitis, but after repeated use a rebound effect may occur, causing the congestion to get worse. Oral decongestants can also speed up your metabolism, adding to the stress caused by rhinitis.

Homeopathy

Homeopathic treatments for hay fever have been proven to be effective in rigorous trials (see page 50). *Arsenicum album* is good for an itchy, runny nose, sneezing and watering eyes. *Gelsemium* curbs repetitive sneezing, a blocked or runny nose and an itchy throat. *Euphrasia* is useful for the relief of red, itchy, watery eyes.

Supplements

Vitamin C acts as a natural antihistamine. Increasing your intake in the months leading up to the pollen season may be an effective preventative measure. It is best to get your Vitamin C from whole foods, such as fruit, peppers and broccoli, but you could try supplements, particularly if you are allergic to citrus fruit.

'Fake' lore remedies

Many people take pollen extract supplements a few months before their worst season to desensitise themselves, but there is no scientific evidence that this works, and it may even be dangerous for a few highly sensitive individuals. The same applies to the folk remedies of local bee pollen and local honey, taken for the same purpose. No beneficial effect has been shown for them, and there is a slim chance that they might be dangerous for sensitive individuals – seek professional advice if you are unsure.

Decongestants
Herbs like fenugreek, nettles, anise and horehound have a natural decongestant action. Half to one teaspoon of liquorice tincture taken in warm water twice daily for five days a week is also recommended by herbalists, although recent reports indicate that this may carry a risk of water retention (swelling of the ankles, fingers and under the eyes). Inhaling eucalyptus vapours from an essential oil or boiling leaves is also excellent for decongestion.

WATER THERAPY

Conventional treatments can have side effects, and many people prefer to rely on natural treatment options. One such alternative is simply water. Properly administered, water can help to decongest your blocked nose and sinuses.

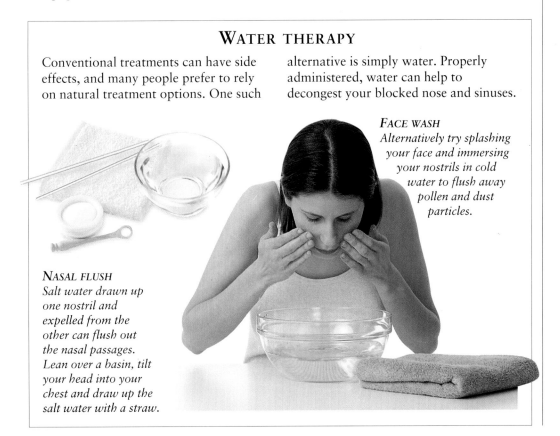

FACE WASH
Alternatively try splashing your face and immersing your nostrils in cold water to flush away pollen and dust particles.

NASAL FLUSH
Salt water drawn up one nostril and expelled from the other can flush out the nasal passages. Lean over a basin, tilt your head into your chest and draw up the salt water with a straw.

ASTHMA

Although asthma usually progresses no further than an irritating or debilitating condition, it can be fatal: over 1500 people die from asthma every year in the UK alone.

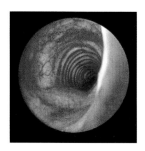

BRONCHIOLES
A view of the inside of a bronchiole shows the rings of smooth muscle which contract during an asthma attack and constrict the airway.

Asthma (or more exactly, bronchial asthma) is a condition where the airways become constricted and filled with mucus. The constriction is caused by the contraction of the smooth muscle within the walls of the bronchi and bronchioles, accompanied by increased mucus secretion. These are reactions to irritation of the sensitive lining of the passages by microscopic particles and vapours, which act as allergens. The allergens provoke an allergic reaction, causing the mast cells of the bronchial linings to release their load of histamines and other inflammatory substances. These mediators cause the constriction of the smooth muscle and excretion of mucus.

SYMPTOMS OF AN ASTHMA ATTACK

Asthma symptoms range in severity from slight shortness of breath, through tightness of the chest, wheezing and dry coughs, to suffocation. The milder symptoms may simply be irritating or uncomfortable, but a severe attack can induce panic and distress. Worsening breathlessness, heavy sweating and a racing heart lead to low levels of oxygen in the blood, which can cause a bluish colour in the face and lips – a condition known as cyanosis.

TRIGGERS OF ASTHMA ATTACKS

The most obvious triggers are the airborne allergens, but there are also non-inhalant triggers. Extreme cold or dryness can irritate the airways of sufferers (see Chapter 7), and exercise is a major risk factor although precautions can help (see page 74).

Food allergy is also linked to asthma. Milk seems to increase its prevalence and severity, and powdery substances like flour, baking powder or ground pepper can act as inhalant irritants. Any food that can cause an allergic reaction (which is potentially all foods) can also cause asthma – usually as a hidden food allergy.

TREATMENT FOR ASTHMA

Medication is the first line of treatment for asthma. Some is preventative, or prophylactic, such as sodium cromoglycate (Intal), or corticosteroid taken through an inhaler. Others are used once an attack has started. These include bronchodilators such as salbutamol, again taken through an inhaler or nebuliser (see page 74). There are many other drugs available, but several of them have side effects (see Chapter 2). Nonetheless, if your asthma is severe you should continue to take your medication as long as you need it.

Reducing your exposure to triggers, following the strategies outlined earlier in the chapter, may make you more comfortable on less medication, or even none.

Although problems arise when exercise is a trigger, there is no need for asthmatics to avoid exercise altogether, as shown by

AFFECTED AREAS IN ASTHMA

The upper part of the airway leading from the mouth to the lungs is known as the trachea. It branches in the chest to become the bronchi, which branch further to become bronchioles, which lead to the air sacs of the lungs. In an attack, the bronchioles become inflamed, and they constrict and produce mucus, causing wheezing and shortness of breath.

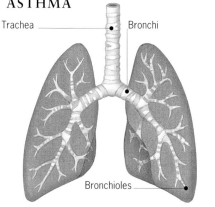

Trachea

Bronchi

Bronchioles

THE LUNGS
The air sacs of the lungs provide a vast surface area over which to exchange waste gases for oxygen.

Treating Asthma with
Natural Remedies

Many asthmatics suffer from mild symptoms, which are irritating but not dangerous. Instead of relying on steadily increasing doses of medication, you could try some natural alternatives to drugs.

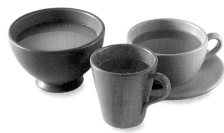

Serious asthma attacks require immediate medical attention, but for milder symptoms – slight wheeziness and shortness of breath – try some of the following natural remedies.

Warm liquids can act as expectorants, making it easier to cough up mucus from the lungs. Half to one cup of a warm beverage like soup, herbal tea or plain warm water every half hour or so relaxes the bronchial muscles. Marshmallow and slippery elm tea have expectorant effects. Passion flower tea can help soothe asthma provoked by tension or nervous conditions.

Deep breathing and warm-up routines will also reduce stress-related asthma. Deep breathing utilises the diaphragm,

EXPECTORANTS
The heat from warm liquids diffuses to the bronchial tubes and dilates blood vessels, relaxing the bronchioles and easing symptoms.

whereas most asthmatics tend to use the shoulder and chest muscles to breathe which only inflates and deflates the upper parts of the lungs.

BREATHING TECHNIQUES

Try this five-minutes-a-day technique developed by the American Lung Association as a preventative routine. Learning to breathe more fully by following these exercises for five minutes every day can reduce the need for therapy from drugs. They can be practised whenever you can find the time and space for a few moments on your own in a quiet, empty room, preferably with a soft surface on which you can lie.

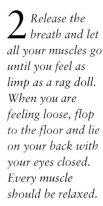

1 *Stand up straight and make all your muscles very tight. Take a deep breath and hold it, point your chin to the ceiling and hold your arms out straight and stiff. Hold this pose for a few seconds.*

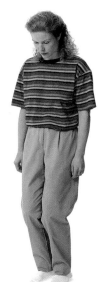

2 *Release the breath and let all your muscles go until you feel as limp as a rag doll. When you are feeling loose, flop to the floor and lie on your back with your eyes closed. Every muscle should be relaxed.*

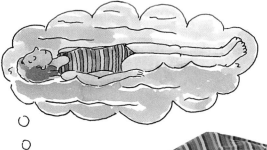

3 *Imagine you are floating down a river. Concentrate on each muscle, sensing how loose they are. Breathe softly, as if you were asleep, and stay quiet. Whenever you feel an attack coming on use this sensation of limpness to help you relax.*

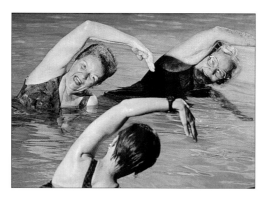

asthmatic athletes like Steve Ovett, a former world record holder. The following steps can help asthma sufferers to exercise safely.

Preventing exercise-induced asthma

Exercising in cold, dry conditions is not advisable, but warm, wet air can soothe the lungs. Swimming is therefore an excellent exercise for asthmatics. There is also some suggestion (from a 1980 study at Yale) that taking vitamin C supplements just before exercise can help relieve wheezing. Wearing a mask can help with activities like running, cycling and skiing, because it keeps out potential irritants, and helps to keep the air reaching the lungs warm and moist.

MAGNESIUM AND ASTHMA

Magnesium deficiency is recognised as an important factor in asthma. Magnesium is essential for muscle relaxation, and a deficiency makes it harder for muscles, such as those around the bronchi, to relax after they contract. This is what happens in an asthma attack, as the bronchial muscles go into spasm – a process known as bronchospasm. In general, an asthma sufferer who is deficient in magnesium is at greater risk of bronchospasm.

A study of 2600 adults in Nottingham, England and in Boston, USA (published in *The Lancet* in 1994) showed that the average diet was deficient in magnesium, and that people with a higher consumption of magnesium had only half of the airway hyper-reactivity of those with the lowest intake. Asthma sufferers should consider having the level of magnesium in their red blood cells (not their serum) assessed by a hospital laboratory. People who are deficient should eat more magnesium-rich foods, such as wholegrain cereals, green vegetables, pulses, apricots and bananas, or they could take a supplement, on the advice of their doctor or nutritionist.

ASTHMA MEDICATION TABLE

This table shows the main medications used to control asthma and provide relief during an attack. With inhalers the doses are low, and so is the risk of side effects. Some people react to the propellant in inhalants. Powder forms do not have propellants but may contain lactose as filler. Turbohalers contain neither.

DRUG TYPE	ACTION	POSSIBLE SIDE EFFECTS	EXAMPLES
Preventers (brown, orange, or red inhalers)	Guard against asthma attacks by making airways less irritable and reducing inflammation	Throat irritation, coughing, thrush (yeast infection). Needs to be taken regularly	Beclomethasone, budesonide, fluticasone
Non-steroid preventers (white, or yellow and green inhalers)	Reduce severity of response to allergens and therefore reduce irritability of the airways	Negligible	Sodium cromoglycate, nedocromil sodium
Short acting relievers (inhalers: blue, or black with light blue writing)	Relieve symptoms quickly in the event of an attack. They open up the airways and increase heartbeat	Tremors, nervous tension, headache, flushing, dry mouth. Over-reliance on these should be avoided	Salbutamol, terbutaline, fenoterol
Slow-acting relievers (inhalers: green or black with yellow writing; white tablets; xanthine tablets)	Provide longer lasting relief in the event of an attack by relaxing the muscles around the airways	Dry mouth, difficulty in passing urine and constipation (at high doses). Xanthines may cause irregular heartbeat and nausea, so require close medical supervision	Oxitropium, salmeterol, xanthines such as theophylline
Corticosteroid tablets	For control of chronic symptoms. They act to make the airways less irritable	Husky voice, weight gain, bone thinning, high blood pressure, water retention. May lead to physical dependence	Prednisolone, prednisone

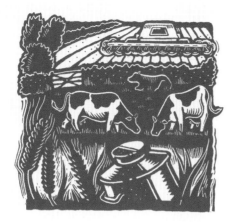

FOOD ALLERGIES

Among the least understood of the allergic reactions are food allergies. Conventional allergists label them intolerances, if they admit that such reactions exist at all. But environmental allergists claim that reactions to food underlie a vast range of both acute and chronic disorders, and that a significant proportion of the population suffers to some degree.

UNDERSTANDING FOOD ALLERGIES

Food allergies fall into two camps. Immediate allergies, which produce symptoms within minutes, and hidden allergies where the cause is not obvious because symptoms are delayed.

THE USUAL SUSPECTS

Commonly implicated foods in immediate food allergy include:

▶ *Eggs*
▶ *Cow's milk*
▶ *Nuts*
▶ *Peanuts*
▶ *Wheat*
▶ *Soya*
▶ *Shellfish*
▶ *Fish*
▶ *Seeds (for example, sesame)*

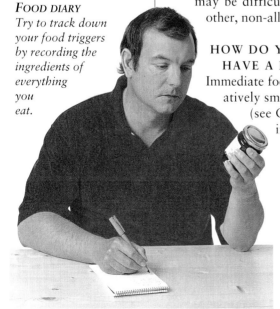

FOOD DIARY
Try to track down your food triggers by recording the ingredients of everything you eat.

The two types of food allergy divide along the lines of Type A and B reactions. Immediate ones are Type A. They produce familiar acute allergic symptoms such as swelling, rashes and itching. Conventional allergists see these as allergies because they have a recognised immunological mechanism – the symptoms are known to be caused by the action of the IgE antibody. A common example of this sort is peanut allergy. Within a few minutes of eating a peanut, someone who is allergic may experience swollen lips and a rash on various parts of their body (urticaria).

In contrast hidden food allergies are Type B reactions. Sufferers have delayed onset of a wide variety of chronic symptoms, and the mechanisms are poorly understood. While immediate food allergies are fairly clear cut, hidden food reactions are far more complicated and seem to be more common. They may be difficult to distinguish from other, non-allergic reactions.

HOW DO YOU KNOW IF YOU HAVE A FOOD ALLERGY?

Immediate food allergies cause a relatively small range of conditions (see Chapter 1) and usually involve a fairly limited list of commonly implicated triggers. You should suspect an immediate food allergy if you notice the rapid onset of symptoms after eating a particular food.

Even when dealing with immediate food reactions, however, it may not always be obvious which food is causing your symptoms. A single, minor ingredient may be to blame. If you cannot readily pinpoint the cause you should try keeping a food diary. Record all the food you eat, including snacks. List all the additives (preservatives, colourings and others) and all the individual ingredients of meals, then try to relate your symptoms to a recurring item. A knowledge of hidden food ingredients may help in this detective work (see page 92).

Associations discovered through keeping a food diary are generally the strongest clues to the culprit. RAST or skin prick tests may help to confirm the sensitivity, but these tests are not 100 per cent accurate. Evidence gained by observation is usually more reliable than tests. The best route is to check whether avoidance of the suspect food item 'cures' the symptoms. If it does, and a subsequent challenge with the food (or eating it by accident) causes reactions, a positive identification is confirmed.

Similar steps may help you to determine whether you have a hidden food allergy. If you have a range of vague and/or chronic symptoms, you should always get them thoroughly checked out by a doctor. However, if proper medical investigation cannot determine the cause of your symptoms, you should consider the possibility that they may be caused by a hidden allergy.

ALLERGIES TO RELATED FOODS

Laboratory tests suggest that closely related foods often share allergens. Blood serum (which contains the tell-tale IgE antibodies that cause immediate food reactions) from people with an immediate allergy to one food will often show evidence of reaction to closely related foods. Such cross-reaction occurs, for example, with members of the legume family, particularly between peanuts and soya beans and with tree nuts such as walnuts, pecans, hazels and brazils. There is also a cross-reaction between grains and between some fruits and vegetables.

Where cross-reactions occur with fruits and vegetables, a link with other forms of allergy is not uncommon – for instance airborne or contact allergies. A whole range of these cross-reactions have been reported, involving dozens of fruits and vegetables. A A person with an immediate food allergy to members of the botanical family Solanaceae (potato, tomato, capsicum, aubergine) might, for example, show evidence of a contact allergy on peeling potatoes.

However, some cross-reactions occur with allergens from plants which are not related. Someone allergic to birch pollen, for instance, may be worse if they eat certain nuts and fruits. In these cases allergists assume that the different plants simply happen to share a similar protein or other molecule which acts as an allergen.

WHY ALLERGIC REACTIONS MAY NOT ALWAYS APPEAR

There are a variety of factors that influence if and when a food causes an allergic reaction. In some cases heating a food may weaken or destroy its tendency to cause allergy – its allergenicity. Conversely, a food might only produce reaction in its cooked form. Other foods become more troublesome after processing – for example, certain fish are more allergenic after canning.

The degree of ripeness of a fruit may affect its allergenicity, as may the effect of processing. In general, ripeness increases allergenicity and processing decreases it. Different varieties of the same food can vary in their allergenicity. This is particularly well documented for potatoes and honey – a sufferer may be allergic to just one variety and be unaffected by eating others.

Sometimes a food allergy only produces symptoms through its effect on another allergy. For instance, food allergies may have a priming effect on inhalant allergies. A hidden allergy to cow's milk may cause little or no trouble for most of the year, but during the pollen season the cow's milk could be a priming agent for hay fever. Excluding cow's milk might therefore alleviate the symptoms of hay fever.

A rare but potentially life threatening condition is anaphylaxis induced by a combination of exercise and eating a particular food (see Chapter 7). Only if both triggers are present does the reaction occur. Known food triggers in exercise-induced anaphylaxis include celery, shellfish, wheat and peaches. In a few cases specific food triggers cannot be identified, but there is still a connection with eating.

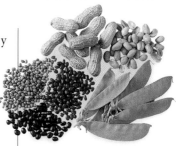

LEGUMES
Peanuts are not actually nuts, but members of the same family as peas and beans – the legumes.

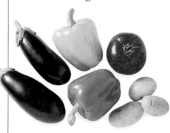

SOLANACEAE
Aubergines, tomatoes, potatoes and peppers all belong to this family.

FOOD ALLERGY RELATED CONDITIONS

Immediate food allergy can cause or complicate many allergic conditions, including problems in parts of the body not obviously associated with eating or digestion.

CONDITION	COMMENTS
Asthma	Immediate food reactions and immediate food additive reactions may be involved in 5-10% of asthmatics
Urticaria ('nettle rash' or 'hives')	10-15% of cases may relate to immediate food allergy
Oral allergy (itching and swelling of lips, tongue and sometimes throat)	Immediate food allergy is involved in the majority of cases
Laryngeal oedema (throat swelling)	Immediate food reactions are often involved
Anaphylaxis (allergic collapse with fall of blood pressure and/or severe wheezing)	Immediate food allergy is a common cause, especially allergy to nuts
Eczema	Elimination diet trials suggest that anyone with persistent atopic eczema has at least a 50% chance of a major contributory food reaction. Although most will be examples of hidden food allergy, some immediate food reactions may also be present
Rhinitis (nasal allergy, including hay fever)	30% of cases may involve food allergy, although most reactions will be hidden rather than immediate

HIDDEN FOOD REACTIONS

When there is a delay between eating a food and the onset of symptoms, it is much harder to pin down the culprit – this is a hidden food reaction.

Masked allergy
If the delay between consuming a food and symptoms is long enough, and the allergenic food is something common, like milk, reactions may start to overlap and become almost continuous. Some of these allergenic foods may actually be addictive, so that consuming them provides temporary relief from symptoms, and avoiding them can cause a withdrawal effect. This phenomenon is known as 'masked allergy'.

Hidden food reactions are the cause of some of the most bitter controversies in the field of allergy research. The controversy centres on whether the reactions are true allergic reactions, or simply types of intolerance.

HIDDEN FOOD ALLERGY

Some intolerance mechanisms are comparatively well understood (see below), but for the majority of delayed onset food reactions encountered the exact mechanism remains unknown. Environmental allergists regard symptoms as probably being caused by food allergy if they are relieved by avoiding the food and provoked by subsequent challenge, provided that there is no evidence that these other mechanisms are involved.

Conventional allergists tend to only accept allergy as a cause of adverse reactions to foods if IgE antibodies are involved (Type I allergy). They tend to overlook the symptoms caused by Type B allergies, or may attribute them to intolerance or psychological causes. But the truth is that in most cases of hidden food reaction the mechanism is not properly understood, so that a definition based on symptoms and response to treatment makes more sense.

CHARACTERISTIC FEATURES OF HIDDEN FOOD ALLERGY

One of the best ways to define 'hidden food allergy' is to explain some of the characteristic features, and the problems they pose for sufferers and practitioners.

FOOD INTOLERANCE

Some reactions to foods are neither immediate allergies nor hidden allergies. These are properly termed food intolerance. A number of intolerance mechanisms have been described – the four main ones are outlined below, with examples of the foods and substances involved in each condition.

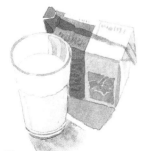

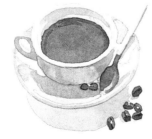

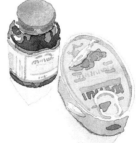

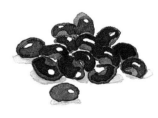

ENZYME DEFECTS
Intolerance can be caused by a defective enzyme, as with lactose intolerance, where the sufferer cannot break down lactose, a sugar found in milk.

PHARMACOLOGICAL EFFECT
This is where intolerance is caused by the direct action of a substance in the food, such as caffeine in coffee. This type of intolerance is similar to the effects of a drug.

INTERACTION WITH A DRUG
Substances in food may interact adversely with drugs, causing intolerance reactions. For instance amines, found in anchovies, may interact with some antidepressants.

TOXINS IN FOOD
This is where an adverse reaction is caused by the toxic effects of a substance in the food, such as lectin in kidney beans which are not properly cooked.

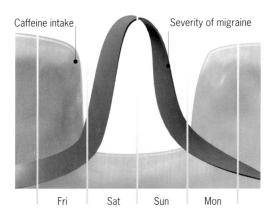

WEEKEND MIGRAINE
As caffeine intake drops at the weekend a withdrawal effect can cause a 'weekend migraine' – a symptom of masked caffeine allergy sometimes experienced by office workers.

Multiple symptoms

Whereas immediate food allergy usually produces a limited range of symptoms, in hidden food allergy it is common for there to be multiple symptoms – typically symptoms will relate to a number of organ systems. Also, most sufferers will be sensitive to more than one food – usually between three and six but sometimes many more.

Symptom pattern

Hidden food allergy symptoms are usually prolonged, but they often fluctuate. The extent to which they do this largely depends on the frequency with which the food is eaten and whether it is eaten in conjunction with other troublesome foods. This variability means that sufferers can almost never deduce the cause of the trouble from the pattern of symptoms.

Withdrawal effects

Even though a food is causing allergic symptoms its deliberate or accidental avoidance may precipitate or worsen symptoms. Obviously this makes it harder for a sufferer to spot his or her trigger food, although an experienced practitioner may look for withdrawal symptoms as a clue. Withdrawal effects do not always occur, however, and the absence of a withdrawal response on avoiding a suspect food is no evidence that the food is not a problem.

Unmasking

Brief exclusion of the trigger food from the diet, followed by reintroduction, will result in a swifter and stronger reaction than before. This is how most practitioners make their diagnoses. This response is most reliably produced after one to three weeks of exclusion, during which time challenging with the food produces an obvious reaction, effectively unmasking the hidden allergy.

Timing of symptoms

In hidden food allergy worsening of symptoms may show no relationship to when foods were eaten. After unmasking, some foods in some patients may cause immediate reactions while others cause symptoms which may be delayed for as long as two days. Most reactions start between 1 to 4 hours after consumption.

Building tolerance

By completely avoiding the trigger food for weeks or perhaps months a sufferer may be able to develop tolerance. Maintaining tolerance depends on remaining below the threshold of consumption frequency and quantity for that person, but this may improve with time and successful avoidance.

Theron Randolph

No discussion of hidden and masked food allergy is complete without mentioning the American allergist Theron Randolph, who was an instrumental figure in the early study of hidden food allergies. By the 1940s he had started the clinical ecology movement, identifying and describing hidden food allergies in a significant proportion of his patients. He was also one of the first to describe masked food allergies, particularly to milk, wheat and caffeine-containing beverages, a pattern he saw among his patients again and again.

CONDITIONS IN HIDDEN FOOD ALLERGY

Common symptoms of hidden food allergy can involve all organ systems of the body – for instance, skin or cardiovascular conditions. Having unrelated symptoms from more than one system can be a telltale clue that hidden food allergy is involved.

ORGAN SYSTEM	COMMON SYMPTOMS
Respiratory	Asthma; rhinitis (nasal allergy); glue ear
Gastrointestinal	Infantile colitis (intestinal disorder causing diarrhoea); infantile colic; coeliac disease (intolerance of gluten in wheat and other cereals); Crohn's disease (chronic inflammation of the intestinal tract); recurrent abdominal pain (especially in children); diarrhoea and constipation; irritable bowel syndrome
Skin	Eczema; urticaria (nettle rash or hives); dermatitis herpetiformis (tiny, itchy blisters)
Central nervous system	Headache and migraine; hyperactivity; mood changes
Cardiovascular	Palpitations (heart rhythm abnormalities)
Musculoskeletal	Joint pain; arthritis; muscle pain
Renal tract	Bed-wetting; nephrotic syndrome (kidney dysfunction); non-bacterial cystitis; chronic interstitial cystitis
Psychiatric	Somatisation disorder (expression of mental and emotional problems as physical disorders); fatigue; hypersomnia (excessive sleeping); insomnia

FINDING HELP FOR YOUR FOOD ALLERGY

Different practitioners vary in their approach to the treatment of food allergies. It is important to understand the different approaches in order to find the right one for your allergy.

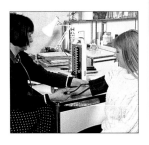

FIRST PORT OF CALL
Your general practitioner should always be the first person you consult. A good GP will be familiar with your history, and thus able to see any new symptoms within the context of previous problems.

There is a confusing range of practitioners working in the field of allergies. But whoever you see, you must be able to trust that your practitioner is safe and well-trained. If you have any doubt don't be afraid to check his or her qualifications, and if possible go through a respected organisation if you are finding a practitioner for yourself.

THE GENERAL PRACTITIONER
Seeing a doctor is an important first step for anyone who thinks they may be suffering from an allergy. This is because it is essential to have a proper medical checkup, by a qualified professional, in order to rule out any other possible causes of your symptoms. On the other hand, a conventional GP's approach to allergies may have some shortcomings.

The lack of a reliable test for hidden food allergy, and the fact that the subject is not generally taught at medical schools, makes it unlikely that most family doctors will consider hidden food allergy when faced with any but the most obvious case. Although the concept is now well recognised (it is known in medical circles as food intolerance), the breadth of related conditions and the range of possible foods involved may be greatly underestimated by many GPs.

For instance, a family doctor might well suggest a simple elimination diet – say, cutting out milk – to deal with an obvious food reaction, but if this did not produce results, he or she might be unlikely to consider other possible triggers.

Doctors are more likely to diagnose a psychological cause for chronic allergic illness without investigating further. They may use the term 'somatisation disorder', to explain cases of patients who exhibit a wide range of apparently unrelated symptoms, where medical tests show no abnormalities. The term means that an illness is caused by psychological distress manifesting itself through the body. While there is no doubt that psychological mechanisms can produce bodily symptoms, there is also strong evidence that many symptoms attributed to somatisation disorder may be due to allergic responses.

A family doctor with a special interest in allergy, may run a diagnosis and advice service, often with the help of a specialist nurse and possibly a dietitian. This sort of service can provide the regular support that a hospital-based practice cannot.

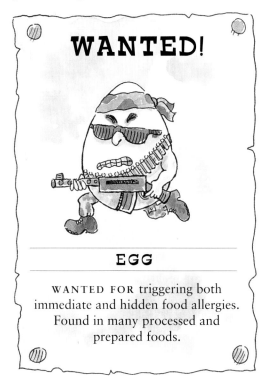

WANTED!

EGG

WANTED FOR triggering both immediate and hidden food allergies. Found in many processed and prepared foods.

THE CONVENTIONAL ALLERGY SPECIALIST

General allergy specialists are rare in the UK, and operate only from hospital-based clinical practices. They are more common in other countries, such as the USA. When making diagnoses, conventional allergists use skin-prick tests and serological tests such as RAST (neither of which are effective for hidden food allergies). They sometimes challenge with food under supervision to confirm immediate allergies. But because they work within the narrow, conventional definition of allergies their interests may extend only as far as straightforward food reactions with a clear immunological mechanism – mainly immediate food allergies.

THE ENVIRONMENTAL ALLERGIST

Also known as clinical ecologists, environmental allergists are fully qualified doctors who have adopted a more holistic, symptom-oriented approach to allergies in general, and particularly to food allergies. For diagnosis they use elimination diets and food challenges, as well as conventional allergists' methods like prick and patch tests. Most will also be concerned about nutrition and may use tests of nutrient levels in blood samples. For treatment they call on a wide range of methods and tools, including drugs, diets, supplements and immunotherapy. They will also consider the role of yeasts and other gut microflora.

Although a few work in hospitals, environmental allergists are regarded as practising outside the mainstream because they emphasise environmental and nutritional factors. Some of their methods have been validated on a scientific basis, but the studies tend to be disregarded by conventional doctors. Other methods have not been properly tested, or may be hard to test, but this does not mean that they are ineffective.

ALTERNATIVE THERAPISTS

While the severe and life-threatening aspects of immediate food allergies need proper medical attention, the gentler, less invasive techniques of alternative medicine may be more suitable for the treatment of hidden food allergies than conventional methods. Homeopathy and acupuncture have good track records in treating some allergies (hay fever and asthma), and naturopathy may be particularly appropriate for food allergies.

VISITING A DIETITIAN

Many dietitians will be aware of both immediate and hidden food allergy, as well as the methods available for their diagnosis. Some will have had training in the use of elimination diets. They can provide valuable advice on how to compensate for the nutritional inadequacies of elimination diets, and help patients through any practical and social difficulties associated with a new diet.

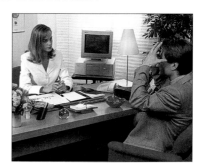

ANALYSING YOUR NUTRITION
A dietitian may use a computer program to devise a balanced, personalised elimination diet.

It is important, however, to check the accreditation of each practitioner. Some complementary disciplines maintain a register of qualified practitioners to try to ensure high standards.

Unfortunately, there can be pitfalls in alternative treatment. Many treatments simply do not work, or what works for one person may be quite ineffective for another, and many of the tests used are unproven. Inappropriate or ill-advised dietary treatments may exacerbate conditions or cause problems of their own. Before consulting an alternative practitioner it is always sensible to have a thorough medical examination first, to make sure that a serious medical condition is not missed.

BE YOUR OWN FOOD TRIGGER DETECTIVE

Testing for immediate food allergies should be carried out only in a medical setting, and treatments will need to be performed by a qualified doctor. However, the essential steps in diagnosing and treating hidden food allergies can all be done at home.

The first step is to keep an allergy diary (see page 44). Once some suspects have been identified you can avoid them to see whether your symptoms improve. If this effectively clears your symptoms the next step is to try a food challenge – by reintroducing the suspect food – to check that it is indeed the trigger.

Unfortunately, hidden food allergies are rarely this clear-cut. Sufferers are usually allergic to between three and six foods, and symptoms will not clear until most or all of

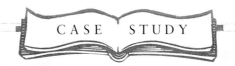

Food Allergy Sufferer

Migraine is a widespread and debilitating affliction which can last for days and seem to strike without reason. The conventional drug treatments on offer may be expensive and ineffective. Food allergies are often the root cause, and a simple elimination diet can trace the triggers and set you on the path to long-term relief.

Jenny is 49 and has suffered from frequent migraine since her teens. The attacks have gradually worsened over the years. She has a severe attack every six to eight weeks where the pain is usually accompanied by vomiting and difficulty in focusing. More often than this she experiences a milder attack which can last for up to four days. Other troublesome symptoms are swollen ankles (oedema) and painful stiff joints. She is overweight despite having good eating habits – her diet consists mainly of vegetable and pasta dishes. Her GP is treating her with drugs, including an expensive one for the worst attacks. She has managed to limit her use of the latter to 24 tablets over the previous three months.

WHAT SHOULD JENNY DO?

Jenny should consider whether food allergy may be the cause of her illness, particularly because of the chronic, drug-resistant nature of her condition. First she should consult an allergist or dietitian. Following their guidance she should keep a food diary for a couple of weeks (see page 44), and then start a strict elimination diet (along the lines of the Stone Age diet – see page 84). If this succeeds in clearing her symptoms she should go on to try food challenges to isolate and identify her potential migraine triggers. By keeping careful records, noting down all the foods she ate (including any added ingredients) and monitoring her symptoms she should be able to find the culprits.

HEALTH
Migraines cause pain and stress, and can be incapacitating. Expensive drug treatment may not be effective, and may have side effects.

DIET
Frequently eaten foods can cause persistent and debilitating conditions. Migraine is a classic symptom of food allergy, as are fluid retention and weight problems.

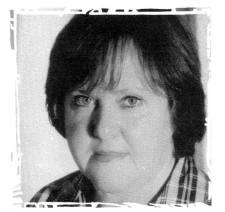

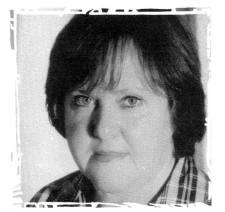

EATING HABITS
Two or more foods could be acting as triggers, the effects of each one masking the effects of the others.

Action Plan

HEALTH
Control the condition through diet, and cut out the need for medication.

DIET
Make a chart of symptom frequency, and use it to trace the effects of a strict elimination diet followed by food challenges.

EATING HABITS
Once challenges have identified the trigger foods, avoid them completely, but make sure to compensate for any nutritional deficiencies by eating a balanced diet and taking supplements.

HOW THINGS TURNED OUT FOR JENNY

Jenny had an initial severe attack at the start of her diet, but then her migraines cleared. After nine days, she started a programme of food challenges, and identified four foods that triggered her migraines. They were wheat, corn (maize), yeast and mushrooms.

By strictly avoiding her triggers, Jenny has not had a headache for three months. She is more relaxed and active, and her other health problems have disappeared.

them have been excluded. The most effective way to do this is to follow the 'Stone Age diet' (see page 84), which, if followed properly, cuts out almost all the most likely food, drink and additive triggers.

FOOD CHALLENGES

A clear and convincing improvement in your symptoms after following the Stone Age diet for up to two weeks is the signal to start testing individual foods. This sort of testing, known as food challenging, is the only sure way to prove that a hidden food allergy is responsible for your symptoms. No one who has severe asthma, however, or who has had serious reactions to food in the past, should attempt challenges without medical supervision.

How to challenge

Food tests should be carried out once a day, at breakfast or lunchtime. The test food can be eaten either on its own, or together with allowed or already tested foods. The test food should then be eaten again with the evening meal, unless a reaction has already occurred. Do not move on to the next food, until you are quite sure you have not reacted – be aware that symptoms may be delayed (especially with grains like wheat, corn and rice), so wait for 24 hours. If you do have a reaction, allow at least 24 hours after your symptoms have substantially improved before moving on to the next food.

Keep a record chart of your tests. If unsure about a reaction, retest it later but make sure that you only test foods that you have avoided for at least five days.

Interpreting your records

Challenging with one food per day may give clear cut results – headache, diarrhoea, an itchy nose, gaining a kilogram (2 lbs) are all tell-tale symptoms. Even apparently minor complaints – poor sleep, irritability or simply feeling unwell – should be regarded as reactions.

But sometimes the picture is unclear. If you felt unwell in the morning, but carried on testing and then got worse, was this due to yesterday's food or today's? Both foods must be retested after at least five days abstinence. If most foods seem to be causing problems you may simply be a slow responder, and are not allowing enough time

between challenges. Go back on the diet until you feel better, and then challenge again more slowly, taking two or three days (or longer) over each challenge.

Complications

Remember, you may feel better on an elimination diet simply because you are doing something about your problem (this is called the placebo effect). To be convincing there should be a clear triggering of symptoms on reintroducing the food or foods. You should also be prepared for much brisker and stronger symptoms than before.

If you avoid a trigger food for weeks or months you may build up some tolerance for it. This can be confusing if you delay testing, but it also means that you may be able to train your body to accept a previously allergenic food, within limits.

TESTING FOODS FOR A CLEAR RESULT

The table below recommends the best forms for testing some of the major hidden food allergens. Individual foods should be reintroduced singly and in a simple form. For example, you should not test bread, as it contains a number of different ingredients. If you reacted after testing bread, you would not know whether it was yeast, wheat or another ingredient (such as soya) that had caused the reaction.

FOOD OR DRINK	TEST FORM
CORN	One fresh or frozen corn on the cob
MILK	Half a pint of full-fat milk
SOYA	A glass of soya milk (check that it is sugar-free)
EGG	One hard-boiled egg and one which is soft-boiled or poached in plain water
YEAST	A quarter teaspoon of fresh baker's yeast mixed in an allowed drink or with allowed food
WHEAT	Two Shredded-Wheat biscuits softened with water or a portion of pure wheat pasta cooked in water
CHOCOLATE	A piece of dark cooking chocolate (should be free of milk and milk solids)
CHEESE	A number of pieces of different types of very pale cheddar (only test cheese if there has been no reaction to milk)
TEA AND COFFEE	A cup of tea or coffee without milk or sugar
CITRUS FRUIT	A selection of wedges of unsweetened orange, grapefruit or lemon

THE STONE AGE DIET

The Stone Age diet is a useful form of elimination diet, because it excludes anything that was not present in the diets of our Stone Age ancestors, more than 10 000 years ago.

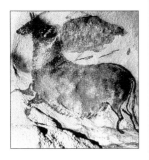

PREHISTORIC PREY
Stone Age art, like this painting from the famous Lascaux cave, dating from 15 000 BC, illustrates the range of prey animals that our ancestors may have hunted.

One theory about food reactions is that allergies and intolerances result from the consumption of foods with which we are not evolutionarily equipped to deal. The introduction of agriculture, and the consumption of foods which are now staples, such as rice and wheat, are all comparatively modern developments. Agriculture and the domestication of animals did not begin until about 10 000 years ago, and changes have speeded up in the past fifty years, with intensive agricultural systems and food manufacture. Our metabolisms and digestive systems, however, have evolved over hundreds of thousands or even millions of years. It may be that the modern diet, rich in foods such as milk and wheat, produces adverse reactions because we are not properly adapted to it.

The Stone Age diet is probably the most comprehensive elimination diet you should follow at home. There are a number of versions of the diet – the following version leaves out cereal grains, sugars, milk and milk products, egg, chicken, citrus fruits, potato, soya, tomato, additives and a number of other possible hidden food allergens. You can customise the diet to meet particular demands – for instance if allergy to fruits is suspected. But do not cut out more than one or two extra foods without medical or dietary advice. The table below lists the main foods you can eat.

The diet should be followed for at least one week, and always for long enough to establish that symptoms have cleared up convincingly. Only if this is successful are foods then reintroduced, one at a time, as

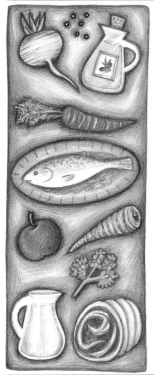

FOODS IN THE STONE AGE DIET

The table below lists the types of foods allowed on the Stone Age diet – these are the foods which would have been available to our Stone Age ancestors. Try to eat organically produced food to avoid possible contamination by pesticides.

FOOD	COMMENTS
Fresh or frozen meat	Any kind including offal
Fresh or frozen fish	Any kind, without batter, breadcrumbs, etc
Fresh vegetables	Any kind except potato, tomato and soya (yam or sweet potato can be substituted for potato)
Fresh fruit	Any kind except citrus fruits (orange, lemon, grapefruit, lime, satsuma)
Grain substitute	Buckwheat, quinoa (a South American grain)
Drinks	Spring water, additive-free juices of allowed fruits, herb and fruit teas (e.g. mint, rosehip)
Seasoning	Sea salt, fresh pepper and herbs
Oils	Olive oil, sunflower oil, safflower oil (avoid unidentified vegetable oil)

food challenges (see page 83), introducing each food for a day only in the first instance. If you suffer from severe asthma, laryngeal oedema, anaphylaxis, schizophrenia or other mental illness (including severe depression), or if you have ever had a severe reaction to any food you should not undertake this kind of testing without supervision.

Keep a chart of your symptoms, starting a week before the diet begins. At the same time keep your exposure to chemicals to a minimum, both in the home and in the workplace. Record your most troublesome symptoms on the chart, and use a scoring system to rate them. Weigh yourself at the same time each day on the same scales (first thing in the morning is best), and record the results. Weight often falls during withdrawal as excess fluid is lost, and may rise suddenly as a reaction to a food. You may need to weigh yourself at night to detect this.

If you normally open your bowels less than once a day, then take Epsom Salts on the first morning of the diet to help clear out your system.

When an elimination diet produces a strongly positive response it is not unusual for there to be marked withdrawal symptoms before the symptoms clear. Typically, withdrawal symptoms commence by the end of the first day or the beginning of the second day, and include headache, aching muscles and fatigue. Often the last withdrawal symptom to clear is weakness and fatigue. In most cases this will have disappeared by the seventh to tenth day of the diet. Take note of any foods you particularly crave or want to avoid, whether or not you experience withdrawal symptoms, as craving or aversion can be a clue to the identity of the trigger foods.

If your usual symptoms normally only occur once a fortnight, or if by the end of a week on the elimination diet you have had no improvement, you should consider

continuing the diet for a further week, especially if you experienced initial withdrawal symptoms but your usual symptoms have not cleared. Work out which two foods you have eaten most frequently on the diet and eliminate these as well for the second week. If you have been constipated during the diet, elimination of troublesome foods from your system may have been slow. In this case, repeat the Epsom Salt mixture on the first morning of the second week.

If your symptoms still do not improve, go back on to a normal diet and seek expert help, as it is possible that you are sensitive to one of the foods in the elimination diet.

Remember, clearing symptoms with an elimination diet is no proof of hidden food allergy. Recurrence of symptoms after eating a food is the best proof and this is where food challenge testing comes in.

Keeping well

Long-term proof comes from staying healthy by avoiding your food triggers. During and after your diet try to eat a wide range of foods, and try not to eat any food frequently. Avoid the foods that caused the worst reactions for several months and eat the foods which provoked minor symptoms no more than once a week – this may help to increase your tolerance.

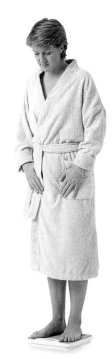

WEIGHING IN
Fluctuations in weight are useful clues. Avoiding your triggers may lead to a rapid weight loss, and positive challenges may cause sudden gains.

WATCH POINTS

In modern life additives are not just found in food. Think carefully about everything you might ingest, and avoid anything that Stone Age man would not have encountered.

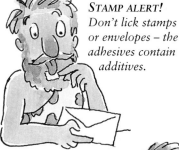

TOOTHPASTE
Use bicarbonate of soda.

STAMP ALERT!
Don't lick stamps or envelopes – the adhesives contain additives.

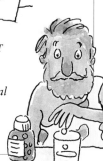

JUST SAY NO
Avoid alcohol and cigarettes – they often cause reactions.

GRIN AND BEAR IT
Medicines contain additives – stop taking non-essential drugs, but check with your doctor.

PREVENTING FOOD ALLERGIES

Very little is known for certain about preventing food allergies, but it seems that protection begins in the womb, and that mothers can influence their children's future food sensitivity.

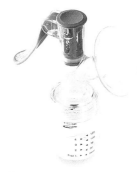

BREAST PUMP
Breastfeeding is very important for good infant nutrition. You can use a breast pump to express your milk, which can be stored in a sterilised container in the fridge or freezer for times when nursing is not convenient.

Genetic factors have a strong influence over the likelihood of developing a food allergy. The prenatal and immediate postnatal environments also seem to play a major role in determining whether an individual becomes sensitised to an allergen. Another important factor is whether your parents were smokers.

AVOIDING EARLY EXPOSURE

Whether or not you develop a food allergy may depend on the foods you ate when you were an infant, and on the foods your mother ate while she was carrying and breast-feeding you.

Transmission of allergens between mother and child

Breastfeeding babies can confer a degree of protection against the development of allergic disease in general. However, substances that the mother eats can be transferred to the baby via the breast milk, and even cross the placental barrier during pregnancy. Prenatal and postnatal infants can therefore be exposed to potentially allergenic foods. This has led to the suggestion that if mothers avoid such foods – especially the main allergy culprits such as nuts, cow's milk and egg – they may help to prevent their children from becoming sensitised. Research is currently under way to test this theory.

The best guidelines at the moment are that the risk of food allergy related illness is reduced if weaning is delayed until after four months of age and if the introduction of common food allergens is delayed until after 12 months of age. Mothers should be aware of hidden allergens – for instance, peanut can be an ingredient of supplements, nipple-soothing creams and oils for premature babies' skins. Try to make sure that an infant does not come into contact with peanuts in any form for the first three years.

AVOID ADDITIVES AND CONTAMINANTS

Substances like food additives and contaminants (toxins and pollutants which we unintentionally consume) may also provoke adverse reactions in some individuals. For instance, they have been proved to provoke asthma in sensitive patients.

Subtract the additives

As with allergenic foods, infants are the most at risk, and pregnant mothers should particularly avoid processed foods which are high in additives. The same applies to everyone – eating fewer additives and avoiding contaminants can only help to decrease the chances of developing any form of sensitivity to them.

ENJOY THE RIGHT FOODS

Children tend to eat lots of sweets and junk food, which expose them to additives. Try to present healthy foods in fun ways to encourage children to eat a better diet.

THE GOOD, THE BAD AND THE ADDITIVE
Avoid food additives, artificial colourings and don't introduce babies to eggs, fish, wheat, nuts, peanuts or cow's milk until they are over one year. Encourage your child to eat fruit, vegetables and fresh meat.

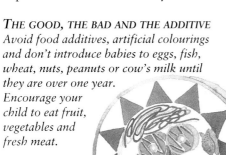

COMMON FOOD ALLERGENS

While any food could potentially cause intolerance or an allergic reaction, the majority of food allergies involve just a handful of particularly troublesome, and often common foods.

Why should some common foods be particularly troublesome? It is probably precisely because they are so common that they cause so many problems – the more we are exposed to a food, the more likely we are to develop a sensitivity to it.

MILK

Milk can cause both immediate and hidden food allergies, and most patients who react to milk suffer from more than one condition or symptom. Milk also causes symptoms in lactose intolerance, where an individual lacks enough of the enzyme needed to break down lactose, the type of sugar found in milk. Intolerance of lactose can cause some symptoms similar to those caused by food allergies (see page 78).

Milk from cows, goats and sheep shares several common allergens, and most people who cannot tolerate cow's milk also react to goat's or sheep's milk. However, some allergic individuals can tolerate a little evaporated milk. Sufferers should try to avoid milk in all foods, and choose substitutes instead (see page 92).

CHEESE

Cheese can cause nearly all the same conditions as cow's milk. It may contain colourings and nuts or other added solid foods and is also generally high in certain chemicals called amines (for example, tyramine), sensitivity to which can cause migraine headache in susceptible individuals. Cheese has lower levels of lactose than milk, making it safer for lactose intolerant people.

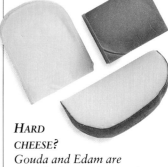

HARD CHEESE?
Gouda and Edam are virtually lactose free, and are safe for most lactose intolerant people. Norwegian Gjetost is a brown cheese made from whey and thus contains no casein, the protein that most milk-sensitive people react to.

DOES IT MATTER WHAT THE COWS EAT?

Does the food of the cow affect the response to its milk? In 1925 the German physician Rohrback reported, 'I have... never failed to enquire as to the feeding of the dairy herd, and have had great satisfaction in observing many a seriously sick infant become normal in a short period, if the offending food was eliminated from the diet given to the dairy cattle'. Ragweed pollen allergy, for instance, might be made worse by milk from cows fed on ragweed but no research has been carried out to confirm this.

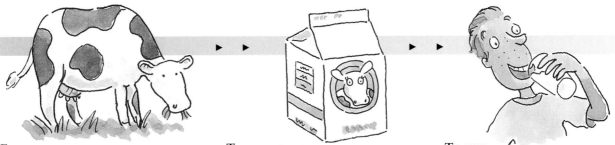

FROM THE COW...
Cows eat both grass and weeds – plants whose pollen is frequently associated with hay fever.

TO THE CARTON...
Could allergens from these pollens pass from the cow's digestive system into the milk...

TO YOU
...and cause an allergic reaction in people who are allergic to those grass and weed pollens?

DIFFERENT GRAINS
Wheat is the most common problem grain. Other grains like oats may serve as a substitute, but loaves may still be dusted with wheat flour.

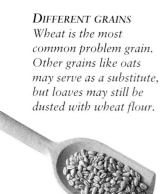

Wheat
Common
hidden food allergen.

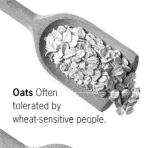

Oats Often
tolerated by
wheat-sensitive people.

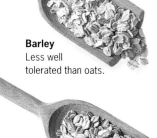

Barley
Less well
tolerated than oats.

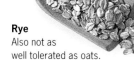

Rye
Also not as
well tolerated as oats.

CHOCOLATE

Chocolate is also commonly blamed for migraine. As with cheese, this may be because of its moderately high amine content. However, the same patients may find that other foods with a higher amine content do not act as migraine triggers, while other foods with negligible amine content, such as milk, do. Even those patients who have a major problem with cheese and chocolate rarely become migraine-free simply by avoiding them – other foods are usually involved, too.

EGGS

Immediate food allergy to eggs is relatively common in small children, often occurring the first time an infant eats egg. It may take the form of a simple rash on the face, or there may be associated swelling of the lips or face. In severe cases there may be wheezing or throat swelling. Delayed reactions to egg may be less common, but children with eczema sometimes show a worsening of their symptoms lasting several days, starting several hours after eating egg.

Egg appears to be a common trigger of hidden food allergy in both children and adults. It can cause a similar range of problems to those caused by milk. Sufferers should avoid egg in all foods, and choose substitutes instead (see page 92), although some find that they can tolerate eggs which are well-cooked – for instance, hard-boiled.

WHEAT

Grains of wheat contain a complex of proteins collectively known as gluten which give wheat its dough-forming properties. In the 1930s this substance was identified as being the cause of coeliac disease, a condition that commonly develops in childhood with a number of symptoms relating to poor digestion and poor absorption of food. Other foods (notably rice and soya) have been shown to produce a similar condition. As well as causing coeliac disease, wheat is probably the commonest hidden food allergen in the UK.

Wheat also causes all the typical hidden food allergy conditions either alone or in combination with other foods. These more widespread effects may be caused by a part of the wheat grain other than the gluten – the bran for instance. Some patients with irritable bowel syndrome who have been taking extra bran on medical advice appear to be much improved when rice or oat bran is substituted and they remove wheat from their diet.

Gluten-free foods

Most food which is labelled as gluten-free is also free from wheat, rye and barley – the other gluten-containing grains. Unfortunately, some packaged food claims to be gluten-free while containing wheat from which the majority of gluten has been removed. It may therefore be unsuitable for a wheat-intolerant individual. Also, it appears likely that coeliac patients may be affected by these so-called 'gluten-free' products. Apart from this confusion over labelling it may not always be obvious that a processed food contains wheat. A wheat intolerant individual should therefore take advice from a dietitian, and read labels very carefully.

Wheat substitutes

Oats are often tolerated by the wheat-intolerant patient, whereas rye and barley are often not. The question of whether oats are tolerated by all coeliac sufferers remains unclear, although many appear to do so. To be safe, wheat-sensitive patients should avoid grains in all foods until they have found which ones are safe for them, choosing substitutes instead (see page 92).

CORN

If wheat is the commonest hidden food allergen in the UK, then corn (historically referred to as maize in the UK) is the most overlooked. It is present in a wide range of manufactured foods as sweetcorn, corn flour, cornflakes, popcorn, corn starch and

WHAT'S IN A WHEAT GRAIN?

Different parts of the grain may cause problems for different people. Some patients report that they are more upset by the bran (the outer husk of the grain), than by the kernel (the central meat of the grain).

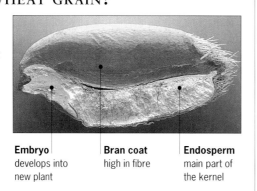

Embryo
develops into
new plant

Bran coat
high in fibre

Endosperm
main part of
the kernel

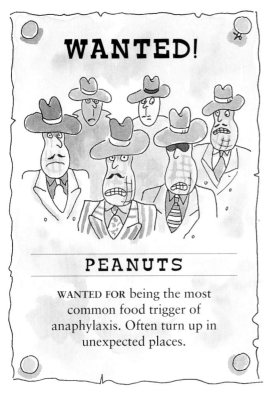

WANTED!

PEANUTS

WANTED FOR being the most common food trigger of anaphylaxis. Often turn up in unexpected places.

corn-derived sugars (glucose, dextrose and others). Early investigators of food allergy tended to be primarily concerned with proteins, and the allergenicity of the carbohydrate parts of foods (the sugars and starch) has been largely overlooked. One problem is that corn has often been used as a substitute for wheat in elimination diets, giving false negative results. In fact, most manufactured foods prepared for wheat intolerant patients contain corn.

As with wheat, the presence of corn in manufactured foods is not always obvious and it is worth consulting a dietitian.

YEAST

Yeast and yeast-containing foods have been shown to be capable of causing urticaria in adults. Avoiding yeast clears up the condition and challenging with brewer's yeast or ingesting the 'thrush' yeast *Candida albicans* causes a recurrence. Other patients with chronic urticaria appear to clear when given anti-yeast diets and nystatin, taken by mouth. This suggests that their urticaria may be due to sensitivity to natural yeasts (including *Candida*) present in the gut.

A much wider role for yeast sensitivity has been suggested. It is claimed that some patients with multiple symptoms, including chronic fatigue and exhaustion, headaches, abdominal pain, bloating and urinary

symptoms, improve substantially on a diet low in yeast and sugars, sometimes coupled with a course of anti-yeast therapy. This theory remains unproved at present.

SHELLFISH

These are a common cause of immediate food allergies, but can also cause hidden allergies. People's reactions to shellfish vary in severity. One reason is that many shellfish are treated with a preservative called benzoate to which some people are allergic or intolerant – different batches of shellfish will have different levels of benzoate.

Anyone who has had an adverse reaction to shellfish should be extremely careful about eating them again, and should be aware of dishes which might contain them, such as paella or jambalaya. Shellfish allergy can cause anaphylaxis.

NUTS

One of the more common triggers for severe immediate food allergy is peanut (also called groundnut), and some people are also allergic to other kinds of nuts (tree nuts). As with shellfish the reasons for this cross-reactivity are unclear, since many nuts belong to unrelated families.

Why do peanuts cause such severe reactions?

One factor may be that they contain lectins, highly toxic compounds that can have direct effects on mast cells (known as pseudo-allergic reactions). Peanuts are not actually nuts at all; they are a member of the legume family, and other legumes contain lectins as well. Some people who are allergic to peanuts have cross-reactivity with other legumes like soya.

YOGHURT VERSUS YEAST

A natural treatment for yeast problems is to eat plenty of live yoghurt. This contains a number of species of bacteria, including *Lactobacillus* which is an important friendly gut bacteria. The bacteria from the yoghurt may be able to out-compete and displace unfriendly gut flora such as yeast. Check that the yoghurt you are buying really is live by following this simple procedure: boil two cups of milk and allow it to cool. Add a teaspoon of the yoghurt and keep the mixture in a sealed vacuum flask for about seven hours. If the original yoghurt was live, the bacteria it contained will have converted the milk into more yoghurt.

LIVE AND KICKING
If you cannot tolerate yoghurt, there are commercial preparations of bacteria available.

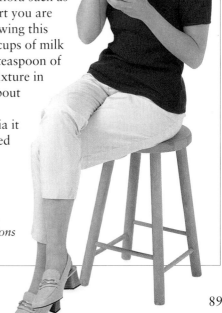

Hypo-Allergenic Cooking with

Healthy Recipes

Egg, yeast and wheat are commonly added to processed foods, and are staple ingredients in many dishes. But there are ways to avoid using them which can allow you to make a variety of tasty, healthy meals.

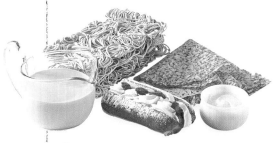

OMNIPRESENT EGGS
Eggs are found in most baked goods, meringue, icing, mayonnaise, salad dressings, noodles, battered and crumbed foods and tinned soups, so it can be difficult to avoid them.

Many people react with horror on being told they will have to cut out ubiquitous foods like egg, yeast and wheat from their diets. However, many common dishes, such as pasta, mayonnaise and bread, can be made without these ingredients.

Egg-free eating
Eggs are sought after not just for their taste, but also for their cooking properties. Commercial egg substitutes are available but often contain different allergens. The recipes given below for egg-free

---

EGG-FREE MAYONNAISE

300 g/10½ oz silken tofu
1 tbsp mustard
100 ml/3½ fl oz olive oil
50 ml/2 fl oz sunflower oil
1 tbsp white wine vinegar
salt and freshly ground black pepper

■ Place the tofu and mustard in a food processor. Blend until smooth.
■ Mix the olive oil with the sunflower oil, and slowly add half to the tofu mixture in a steady stream while the food processor is running. When the mixture begins to thicken and go pale, add the vinegar and seasoning to taste. Process until smooth.
■ Slowly blend in the remaining oil.
Makes 425 ml/15 fl oz

EGG-FREE SPICY BEEF BURGERS

450g/1 lb minced beef
3 spring onions
1 tbsp parsley
½ tsp ground cumin
salt and freshly ground black pepper

■ Chop the parsley and spring onions coarsely so that there will be recognisable pieces in the finished burgers for an interesting texture.
■ Place all the ingredients in a large bowl and mix until well combined.
■ Shape into four flat, round burgers and grill or fry for 8-10 minutes, turning very carefully once during cooking. If frying, heat a little oil in the frying pan first.
■ Serve the burgers in wholemeal pittas filled with mixed salad leaves as a delicious, wheat and yeast free alternative to the more usual bread bun.
Serves 4

EGG AND WHEAT-FREE CRÈME FRAÎCHE SAUCE

1 medium potato, peeled and diced
2 cloves garlic
125g/4½ oz low fat crème fraîche
1 tbsp basil, chopped
salt and freshly ground black pepper

■ Boil 500 ml/18 fl oz water, add the potato and garlic, and simmer for about 12 minutes, or until the potato is tender.
■ Transfer the potato, garlic and half the cooking liquid to a food processor and blend until smooth.
■ Add the crème fraîche and blend.
■ Return the mixture to the pan. Stir in the basil, salt and pepper to taste and cook over a moderate heat until bubbling and thick enough to coat the pasta.
■ Serve immediately with corn pasta.
Serves 4

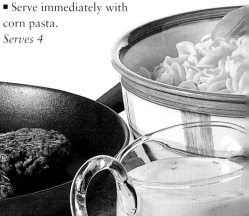

mayonnaise, beef burgers, pasta sauce and ice cream show that it is possible to create a variety of delicious dishes, including some, such as mayonnaise or ice cream, where egg would seem to be an essential ingredient. With simple dishes such as beef burgers, it is relatively easy to avoid common triggers, so long as you make them yourself. However, most people rely on processed versions, which often contain egg and egg derivatives.

Yeast-free eating

If you have a sensitivity to yeast, you must use yeast-free bread like Russian rye, pumpernickel or make your own loaf, such as the soda and corn breads given below, using baking powder as a raising agent.

Some flat breads, such as matzoh or chapati bread, are unleavened, but others, like pitta or nan bread, may have yeast added. You should also avoid alcohol, or at least moderate your intake. The surface of fruit, especially dried fruit, contains small amounts of mould, as do many nuts, and if you have a sensitivity to yeast you should avoid these as well.

Wheat-free eating

Thickeners and fillers are often derived from wheat, which means that a surprising range of foods can cause problems for wheat-sensitive individuals. They need to avoid most processed breads – follow the recipes below to make your own, wheat-free bread. Many

sauces use wheat flour as a thickening ingredient, so a wheat-free pasta sauce is included here to illustrate an alternative option.

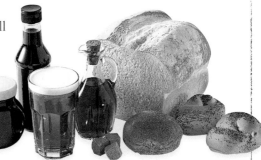

UBIQUITOUS YEAST
Any food or beverage that undergoes fermentation does so due to the presence and activity of yeasts. This includes bread, soy sauce, malt, alcohol, vinegar and many prepared soup stocks.

EGG-FREE RHUBARB YOGHURT ICE CREAM

225 g/8 oz rhubarb, cut into small pieces
2 tbsp soft brown sugar
150 ml/¼ pint whipping cream
500 ml/18 fl oz thick Greek-style yoghurt

■ Place the rhubarb and sugar in a saucepan and add a little water to prevent sticking during cooking. Cook for about 10 minutes, until soft. Allow to cool, then purée the rhubarb.
■ Mix the cream, yoghurt and rhubarb in a large bowl. Add more sugar to taste.
■ Freeze the mixture in a 1 litre/1¾ pint freezer container, uncovered, until thick. Break up any large crystals with a fork. Return to the freezer until frozen.
■ Take the ice cream out of the freezer an hour before serving, to allow it to soften.
Makes 1 litre/ 1¼ pints

YEAST-FREE SODA BREAD

450 g/1 lb strong plain white flour
2 tsp sugar
1 tsp bicarbonate of soda
1 tsp salt
1 tsp cream of tartar
300 ml/½ pint milk

■ Preheat the oven to 190°C/375°F/Gas mark 5.
■ Sieve the flour and dry ingredients into a large bowl.
■ Mix to a soft dough with the milk, adding extra if required.
■ Smooth the dough by gently kneading it and shape into a circle 3.5 cm/1½ inches thick.
■ Put the dough on a greased baking tray and score a large cross over the top
■ Bake for 40 minutes.
Makes 1 loaf

YEAST AND WHEAT-FREE CORN BREAD

175 g/6 oz corn meal (polenta)
25 g/1 oz soya flour
25 g/1 oz oatmeal
3 tsp baking powder
½ tsp salt
2 eggs, beaten
250-300 ml/9-10 fl oz soya milk
1 tbsp melted butter/margarine

■ Preheat the oven to 190°C/375°F/Gas mark 5.
■ Grease a square cake tin 20 cm × 20 cm (8 in × 8 in).
■ Mix the dry ingredients together. Add the eggs, milk and butter or margarine and mix until smooth.
■ Pour the mixture into the prepared tin and bake for approximately 30 minutes.
Makes 1 loaf

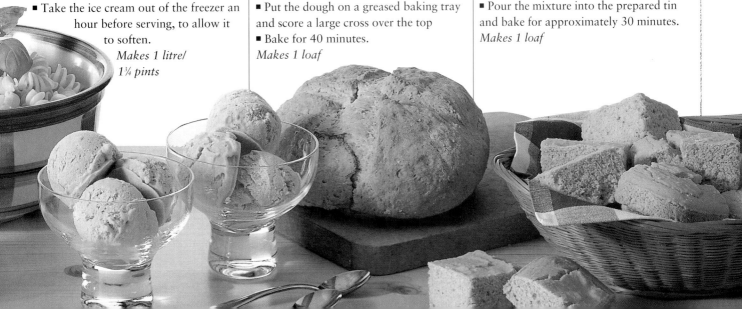

FOODS CONTAINING WHEAT, MILK AND EGG – AND SUBSTITUTES

Avoiding the most common food allergens can be a tall order because they feature so heavily in the Western diet. They are particularly common in processed foods, where they are often difficult to spot. This chart shows you what to look out for, and suggests alternatives that might be suitable.

TYPE OF FOOD	FOODS THAT CONTAIN WHEAT, RYE AND BARLEY	FOODS THAT CONTAIN MILK	FOODS THAT CONTAIN EGG	SUBSTITUTES
Bakery goods and flours	Bread, rolls, scones, fruit loaf, biscuits, cake, wheat, rye or barley flour, malt, cake and pastry mixes	Some biscuits, cakes, breads, and cake and pastry mixes	Some breads and rolls (especially glazed), most cakes and biscuits and mixes, croissants	Breads and bread mixes which are wheat, milk and egg-free, plain rice cakes, cornflour, rice, potato or soya flour, cornmeal, polenta
Pasta and soups	Spaghetti, pasta, noodles, soups thickened with flour, barley or noodles, croutons	Some pasta sauces, creamed soups	Some pastas, egg noodles, noodles in some soups	Rice noodles, pure buckwheat pasta, clear soups without noodles
Cereals	Most including bran, wheat germ, most muesli, some porridge oats contain added wheat (especially 'own label' brands)	Prepared porridge, milk added to cereals		Cornflakes, rice cereals wheat-free porridge oats, wheat-free muesli, (use cereals with fruit juice or milk substitute)
Puddings and sweets	Custard powder, white sauce, pies and pastries, pre-prepared sweets and pudding mixes, pancakes and batters, waffles, fruit crumbles, many sweets and candies, ice-cream cones	Custard, custard powder, white sauce, pies and pastries, sponge and suet puddings, ice cream, milk chocolate, most plain chocolate, sweets with chocolate	Pancakes, batters, pre-prepared pudding mixes, egg custard, soufflés, waffles, meringue, pavlova, doughnuts, marshmallows, ice creams, 'dolly mixtures', Opal fruits	Fruit, special recipe cakes, sweets and pastries, wheat-free batters made with alternative flours, boiled sweets
Vegetables and salads	Avoid sauces, breadcrumbs or gravies served with vegetables or salads	Those prepared with sauces or butter, some gravies and salad dressings	Scrambled and hard-boiled egg added to salads, salad dressings	All fresh, frozen or canned vegetables, all salad foods
Meat and meat products, fish and fish products	Sausages, salami, flour used in thickening gravies and sauces, breadcrumb or batter coatings, hamburgers, pies, pasties, pizza, stuffing, fish cakes, fish fingers, fish in sauce or batter	Dishes cooked in butter, white sauce, milk or cheese, sausages, mortadella, Spam, polony, gravies	Precrumbed foods (for example, fish), hamburgers and sausages, tartar sauce, meat loaf, béarnaise and hollandaise sauces	All fresh fish, meat, most precooked meats if free from binders or stuffing, batters made from alternative flours, alternatives to breadcrumbs (e.g. crushed cornflakes)
Beverages	Malted or barley-containing drinks, root beer, whisky, beer and lager	Chocolate drinks, malt drinks, some tea and coffee whiteners	Ovaltine, some instant coffees, some wines are cleared with egg white	Tea, coffee, cocoa, fruit cordials, soft drinks, mineral water
Milk products	Commercial milk drinks, custard made with custard powder, white sauce, cheese sauce, ice cream with biscuit pieces or sauces	Milk, cheese, butter, most margarine, ice cream, milk powder, yoghurt, buttermilk, condensed or evaporated milks	Some ice creams	Milk substitutes, tofu, vegetable puree (substitute for milk or egg), milk (and whey) free margarine
Ingredients of packet and canned foods	Wheat starch, wheat flour, gluten, wheat gluten, starch, food starch, wheat germ, bran	Milk solids, skim milk, whey, milk proteins, non-fat milk, casein, caseinate, lactose	Vitellin, ovovitellin, livetin, ovomucin, ovomucoid, albumin	Check all packaged foods are free from items listed
Miscellaneous	Baking powder, malt vinegar, some soy sauce, communion wafers, pepper powder		Baking powder	Wheat and egg-free baking powder, wine or cider vinegar, wheat-free soy sauce

FOOD ADDITIVES AND CONTAMINANTS

Additives and contaminants have the potential to cause a wide range of allergic reactions, but can be avoided as organic and additive-free options become increasingly available.

The additives and contaminants in today's food derive from a bewildering array of sources. Agricultural, industrial, traffic and domestic pollution as well as food processing and manufacture, all add inorganic, artificial and natural substances to the things we eat and drink.

CONTAMINANTS AND POLLUTION

Agriculture is the main source of food contaminants in our daily diet. Modern farming methods rely heavily on fertilisers and pesticides. Vast quantities of nitrates, phosphates and other chemicals are added to the soil, accumulating in the produce grown in it and inevitably polluting the water that runs off it. Levels of nitrates and other pollutants in tap water are a serious problem throughout the developed world.

Pesticides

Farmers in Britain use over 400 different pesticides, which fall into three classes: insecticides, fungicides and herbicides. Nearly all of these can be dangerous to humans in their active state, but in theory they are sprayed onto crops long enough before harvesting to degrade before they reach the supermarket shelves. In practice, low levels of pesticides are detected in many foods sampled. In some cases, such as potatoes, pesticides may be sprayed onto food after harvesting.

Other contaminants

Other agricultural pollutants include the antibiotics and hormones fed to farm animals and farmed fish to make them grow faster, larger and leaner. How many of these persist in the meat and fish that reaches the dining table is not clear, nor is the effect they might have. Other sources of pollution affect tap water – for instance drugs from sewage and heavy metals from industry. In one city in the US low concentrations of over 2000 chemicals were detected in the public water supply. Domestic sources of contamination include detergents from washing-up liquids and other cleaners, and organic chemicals from cling film, which may be carcinogens (cancer-causing agents).

Are you in danger?

The food that you eat probably contains only the merest traces of contaminants, but it is impossible to be sure. What's more, it is not really known how bad for you such

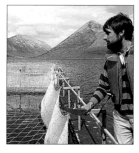

FARMED FISH
Fish farms supply an increasing proportion of the fish in our diet. At some farms fish are fed heavy doses of antibiotics to fight disease.

AVOIDING CONTAMINANTS

Obviously the safest option is to try to avoid contaminants altogether. To achieve this you must buy organic produce and drink bottled or filtered water. Alternatively, investigate different supermarkets to see if they have a policy on testing foods for contamination – some of the big chains set their own limits. Also, simple measures like thorough washing, peeling and cooking can reduce the level of pollutants in the final meal produced.

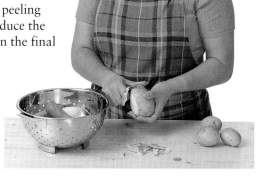

KEEP 'EM PEELED
Many contaminants are concentrated in or restricted to the skins of fruits and vegetables.

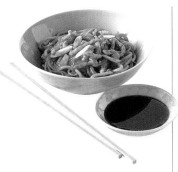

CHINESE RESTAURANT SYNDROME
Monosodium glutamate (MSG) and its relatives, E620-623, are widely used as flavour enhancers. Large amounts of MSG are said to produce a characteristic allergic or intolerant syndrome, although the description of the symptoms involved varies. The use of MSG is particularly associated with food prepared in Chinese restaurants, hence the name of the syndrome. The symptoms include hot flushes, tightness and pain in the chest, headache and even fainting. Although MSG has been reported to trigger attacks in some asthmatics and other symptoms, the latest evidence suggests it might not in fact be responsible for Chinese restaurant syndrome. Other ingredients, such as fermented soy sauce, are now suspected.

traces might be. New chemicals are exhaustively tested, but there are plenty of old ones (still in use here or in the Third World) which were never properly tested, or are, in fact, known toxins or carcinogens.

The extent to which contaminants cause allergic reactions is also unclear but some cases are known: antibiotics in meat have caused allergic reactions, and high levels of nickel and other pollutants in tap water have caused eczema and hives.

ADDITIVES

There are over 3500 different forms of additive found in modern foodstuffs. This includes many natural substances, and it may be only a tiny minority that pose any risk to health. But additives can be found in practically anything that you consume, including many medicines, and allergic or intolerant people should be aware of the variety of guises in which they might meet a trigger additive.

Natural additives

Modern commercial preparation of foods makes it increasingly difficult to be sure that a particular food does not contain a particular ingredient. Some of the most common allergy triggers are some of the most common additives. For example, derivatives of wheat and corn (maize) are commonly used as thickeners and binders in a range of savoury foods. To provide sweetening, sugars and syrups from cane, beet and (most commonly) corn are used. In addition foodstuffs are used as thickeners and sweeteners in liquid medicines and as an apparently inert base for tablets.

Preservatives and flavourings

Preservatives are added to many commercially produced foods to slow their deterioration and are important in the prevention of food poisoning caused by bacterial contamination. They are essential to the modern way of processing, packaging and transporting grocery goods. Fresh foods without preservatives (remember that sugar and salt are preservatives) have to be eaten within a limited period to avoid the risk of microbial contamination. Alternative ways of prolonging storage times include canning, freezing, freeze drying and bottling. Antioxidants prevent degradation of fats and fat-soluble vitamins. Without them fats go rancid.

A number of flavourings and flavour enhancers are now added to foods. Perhaps the most notorious is the enhancer monosodium glutamate, but flavourings like allyl alcohols are also known to be toxic (although they are used in minute amounts). Other food additives include emulsifiers, stabilisers and a wide range of sweeteners and thickeners.

While it is possible for any food additive to cause a problem in a sensitive individual, it appears that some can cause more problems than others. Those approved by the EC are identified by an 'E-number', but not all additives have these (flavourings, for instance, are not classified in this fashion). A few E-numbered additives are the subject of particular controversy, and the main allergy offenders are detailed below.

Antioxidant preservatives

The preservatives with the numbers E320 and E321 are used to preserve oils and fats. They are widely found in commercially prepared packaged foods which contain fats and oils, and trigger asthma, urticaria and other symptoms in susceptible subjects.

Sulphite preservatives

Sulphites (E220 to E228) occur naturally in the fermentation of yeast. Some are therefore always present in wines and beers, and extra ones may be added to beers, wines and fruit juices. They are often used in the preparation of seafood, gelatine, dehydrated vegetables, pickles, preserved meats, sausages, fruit salads, dried fruit and green salads. Sulphites may be sprayed onto prepared foods to preserve them (for example in salad bars and restaurants).

Sulphite sensitivity can be very difficult to detect, or even to suspect. Nonetheless, susceptible asthmatics may react to sulphite when a sulphite-containing food is eaten.

DRIED FRUITS
Some dried fruits have very high levels of sulphite preservatives.

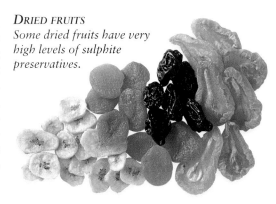

Natural Pest Control

Pests can easily blight your efforts to grow organic produce, but you don't have to rely on synthetic, and often toxic, chemical pesticides. Try using natural pest control methods which will keep away bugs without contaminating your food.

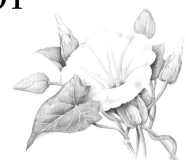

Natural pest control methods, such as friendly insects (e.g. ladybirds), moth-repellent lavender, or aphid-killing infusions of elder leaves can substitute for chemical pesticides. There are several plant remedies you can use to fight pests and diseases. Derris powder from derris root, for instance, controls crawling insects, like ants, while pyrethrum (from pyrethrum daisies) kills leafhoppers, aphids and whiteflies. An infusion of elder leaves also kills aphids. Walnut leaves boiled in water can be used as an ant repellent, while sprays of rosemary or lavender repel moths.

These remedies do have limitations – they do not generally last for more than a day, they only treat the surface of plants, and they may be indiscriminate in the insects they kill.

A lasting method for repelling aphids is to grow French marigolds among your other plants, especially broad beans – marigolds attract hoverflies which prey on the aphids.

Slugs should be removed by hand as they appear in the evening but you should encourage insects like centipedes, spiders, ladybirds, lacewings and hoverflies in your garden as they eat pests like aphids.

Weeding out pests
Avoiding herbicides and chemical weedkillers gives irritating and invasive weeds like bindweed a chance to take hold. Bindweed spreads quickly and winds itself around the stems of plants. Uproot and burn it wherever you find it.

COMPANION PLANTING

Companion planting involves using the proximity of a plant that is offensive to certain insects to protect other plants from their unwelcome attention. These protective plants and herbs are often strong smelling and colourful. Follow a few of the companion planting suggestions below and watch your vegetable garden flourish free from pests.

▶ *Nasturtiums should be planted with your brassicas, broad beans and tomatoes in order to protect them from whitefly and blackfly.*

▶ *French marigolds will protect tomatoes and broad beans from whitefly and greenfly.*

▶ *Basil will repel all flying insects from your tomatoes.*

▶ *Camomile planted among your onions will improve the yield of the crop. Onions grow faster when camomile is present.*

▶ *Cabbage grubs can be fended off with a little mint planted in your cabbage patch.*

▶ *Rosemary repels carrot fly.*

ELDER LEAF SPRAY FOR APHIDS

1 *In a very large saucepan bring 1½ litres (2¼ pints) of water to the boil. Add 200 g (7 oz) of fresh elder leaves and allow to steep for 10 minutes. Strain the infusion and allow it to cool.*

2 *Fill a clean spray bottle (available from garden centres) with the elder leaf infusion. Cover the whole of your plants in the elder spray, making sure the undersides of the leaves and stalks are thoroughly treated.*

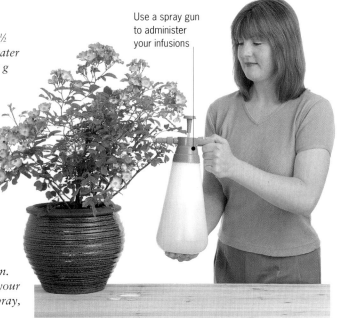

Use a spray gun to administer your infusions

3 *Repeat every day until the aphid infestation has gone. For best results a fresh infusion should be made for each treatment. Regular treatment will keep pests away.*

READING A FOOD LABEL

It is often difficult to identify all the ingredients listed on a food label. Below is a food label such as one might find on a packet of instant noodles together with an explanation of potential hidden allergens.

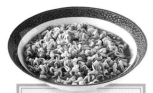

INSTANT NOODLES
INGREDIENTS

Noodles, starch, maltodextrin, caramel, flour, salt, hydrogenated vegetable oil, hydrolysed vegetable protein, beef fat, yeast extract, flavour enhancer (E621), flavourings, emulsifiers, lecithin, albumen, antioxidant (E320)

▶ *Albumen – normally derived from egg.*

▶ *E320: Butylated hydroxyanisole (BHA) – has been implicated as a cause of both urticaria and asthma.*

▶ *Dextrins and caramel – likely to be corn derived.*

▶ *Hydrolysed vegetable protein and lecithin – both usually soya derived.*

▶ *E621: Monosodium glutamate (MSG) – just a few milligrams provoke reactions in sensitive people.*

▶ *Noodles, starch and flour – may all come from wheat. Corn and potato are other possible sources of flour and starch.*

Very susceptible asthmatics may even react to sulphur dioxide fumes from fruit juice or wines to which sulphite has been added. Sulphite sensitivity has also been shown to be a cause of other symptoms such as rhinitis (nasal symptoms) and urticaria.

Nitrate and nitrite preservatives

E249 to E251 are used to preserve and stabilise the colour of some cooked meats (for example ham and bacon) and cheeses. Unfortunately, they have been shown to trigger symptoms such as urticaria and headache in susceptible individuals.

Benzoate preservatives

E210 to E218 are preservatives used in fruit squashes, fruit syrups, fizzy drinks and some medicines. Benzoates also occur naturally in some foods, particularly honey and cranberries. They have been shown to trigger urticaria, possibly asthma and eczema, behavioural effects in some hyperactive children (see page 136) and other symptoms.

Food colours

Azo dyes ('E' numbers 100-180) are commonly found in both foods and medicines, and are among the most problematic additives. They can be broken down by bacteria in the gut to form amines (see page 87). These are absorbed into the bloodstream, and can become bound to proteins in the body, producing both allergic and other biological effects.

Allergies to food dye can be either immediate or hidden. Azo dyes may trigger many symptoms including asthma (affecting about 5 per cent of chronic asthmatics), urticaria (possibly affecting 10-15 per cent of chronic urticaria sufferers), behaviour disturbances, hyperactivity and migraine.

RULES AND REGULATIONS

The use of food additives is governed by regulations which vary from country to country. The labelling of foods containing additives is also regulated.

Problems with labels

Even then there are pitfalls, however. For example, if a patient knows of a sensitivity to a particular preservative (for example BHT, butylated hydroxytoluene, an antioxidant which prevents the degradation of fats) its absence on a food label might reassure.

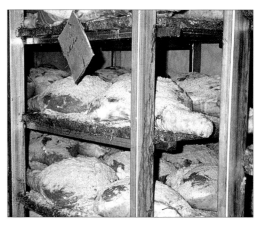

CURE ALL?
The substances now numbered E249 – E251 have been used in the curing of hams and bacon for centuries. However, they can cause urticaria, headache and other symptoms.

But what if one of the labelled ingredients (for example, hydrogenated vegetable oil) had BHT added prior to its purchase by the food manufacturer? The presence of BHT in such circumstances would not be identified on the food label.

Another pitfall involves the words used on the labels. For example, hydrolysed vegetable protein and lecithin may both be derived from soya, but the word soya is unlikely to appear on the label. Peanut is sometimes listed as groundnut or arachis – not knowing that these terms mean peanut could, in extreme cases, be fatal.

Additives in drugs

An even more curious anomaly concerns the lack of labelling requirements for drugs and medicines, both of which commonly contain colourings, flavourings and preservatives. In one survey, 930 out of 2204 drug formulations contained at least one additive.

Are additives your problem?

If you have an unexplained food reaction, the best way to test the possibility that it is caused by reactions to food additives, and not a hidden food allergy to the foods themselves, is to follow a diet which is totally additive free for a few weeks. But you should be aware that food free from overt additives may nonetheless contain residues of pesticides and herbicides. Also, other additives may be added to fresh food to keep it fresh (for example, sulphite may be sprayed onto salads and cut fruits). You may need to try organic foods.

EATING HEALTHILY WITH AN ALLERGY

Restricting your diet to avoid triggering a food allergy need not mean that your nutrition suffers. Many people on anti-allergy diets find that they are eating more healthily than before.

All medical treatments carry some risk of side effects and elimination diets are no exception. Children on restricted diets are at particular risk of malnutrition. Parents have been known to induce nutritional deficiency in their children by going too far with a diet in an attempt to cure their child's allergy. Children are most at risk from reduced protein and energy intake; milk, egg, fish, meat and wheat – the most likely foods to be excluded – are important sources of these nutrients and stunted growth and other signs of malnutrition may result from a lack of them. On the other hand, children with hidden food allergies often have a growth spurt when trigger foods are identified and avoided.

Restricted range of food

The risk of malnutrition in both children and adults results from restricting the range of foods eaten, combined with a failure to compensate for resulting imbalance in the diet. The fewer the number of foods eaten, the greater the risk that the diet will be deficient in one or more individual nutrients (minerals, vitamins, amino acids and essential fatty acids). Nonetheless, it is perfectly possible to maintain excellent nutritional intake while eating a very restricted diet.

A dietitian can help

The dietitian has three useful roles in this context. First, advice can be given on how to avoid specific foods, providing information on hidden sources of allergens. Secondly, analysis of the resulting diet (using a computer for efficiency) can identify what dietary recommendations need to be made to give a good balance of nutrients, using supplements if necessary. Thirdly, suggestions can be given on how to make the diet practical and palatable, bearing in mind that convenience is a major issue in modern domestic catering.

MILK ALLERGY: GETTING SUFFICIENT CALCIUM

The amount of calcium that you really need in your diet is a matter of some debate, as is the degree to which dairy products should provide that calcium. Many races around the world do not consume milk or milk products and yet suffer no greater degree of deficiency than those who do. Neither is it clear what effect milk allergy has on the absorption of calcium and other nutrients from the gut. It is only an assumption that nutrient levels in the bloodstream are reduced by the exclusion of milk.

To be on the safe side, it is best to assume that people from a culture that normally has a high milk intake are at risk from shortage of calcium if they go on a milk-free diet. In particular, it is clear that the needs of growing children and pregnant and lactating women are higher than for other people.

MILK-FREE ZONES
The orange areas on this map show where the majority of adults are lactose intolerant – which includes most of the world's population.

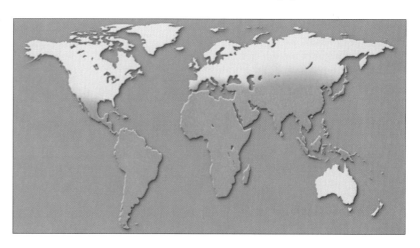

Non-dairy sources of calcium

Going without dairy products does not have to mean going without calcium. There are other foods which can provide this essential mineral, although it is not always well absorbed.

FOOD	CALCIUM (mg per 100 g)	FOOD	CALCIUM (mg per 100 g)
Tofu (steamed and fried)	128	White flour	150
Kelp	1093	Fish paste	280
Tahini paste	140	Spring greens	250
Sesame seeds, hulled	110	Almonds	234
Sardines	550	Fried shrimp	177

Excess or deficiency?

Most patients who start an elimination diet will probably improve their nutrient intake. It is likely that 'antinutrients', such as refined sugar and caffeine, will be reduced; fresher and healthier foods will probably be introduced to the diet; and, by eliminating reactions to food triggers, digestion and therefore absorption will be improved, so that the sufferer can extract more nutrients from what is eaten. On the other hand, it may not hurt to consider the use of a broad hypo-allergenic vitamin/mineral nutritional supplement, but always seek advice as excessive doses of some vitamins and minerals can be dangerous.

On this basis anyone avoiding milk and milk products should compensate with other calcium-rich foods or with supplements. Although calcium-enriched soya milk is rich in calcium, the calcium in other foods may not be well absorbed and special cases such as children (especially in the first year and during puberty) and pregnant or lactating mothers should use supplements. Consult a doctor or dietitian for advice.

Milk and milk products are also an important source of iodine, especially for children. Iodine deficiency (which can depress thyroid function) has been reported in children on an elimination diet, so you should eat other iodine rich foods such as seafood or use iodised salt or get a dietitian's advice on supplements.

NO MIRACLE CURES
Although curing your allergy can help you to lose weight, you will also need to exercise and eat a sensible diet.

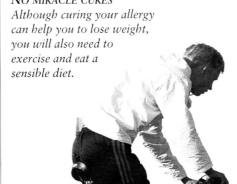

GRAIN ALLERGY: GETTING SUFFICIENT CARBOHYDRATE

Some patients turn out to have a hidden allergy to most or all of the grain foods (wheat, rye, barley, oats, corn, rice). Even if all grains are not involved (for example, some patients can tolerate rice but none of the others), depending too heavily on just one grain can result in nutrient deficiencies.

For patients sensitive only to wheat, wheat-free bakery goods, breads and biscuits are available from specialist suppliers. These are made from other grains, normally corn or rice. Wheat-free pasta, made from corn, rice or buckwheat, is also obtainable. (See page 90 for some wheat-free recipes.) People sensitive to other grains may need to seek alternative sources of carbohydrates – vegetables such as potatoes and yams are a good source of complex carbohydrates, but some important vitamins or minerals may have to be supplemented.

OBESITY AND ALLERGY

It is not unusual to find that elimination of hidden food allergens can act as a most effective weight-reducing diet. Why this should happen is not entirely clear. One possible reason is that a common symptom of hidden food allergy is fluid retention. The marked initial weight loss that occurs in people on elimination diets is almost entirely due to loss of this retained fluid. But this does not account for the sustained weight loss that often occurs.

In some patients the change of diet involves a considerable reduction in calories (if, for example, they were previously eating a lot of foods containing sugar). In others this is not the case, but it may be that improvement in health and well-being leads to an increase in the general level of exercise. This in turn burns off calories and raises an individual's metabolic rate – the rate at which they process calories – decreasing weight further.

It is also possible that in some patients hidden food allergens directly affect their weight regulating mechanism in some way, adversely affecting weight control by a mechanism other than calorie build up. This is a tempting hypothesis for those who fail to lose weight with calorie restriction. However, for non-allergic people, lack of exercise and failure to follow a balanced diet are more likely to be the culprits.

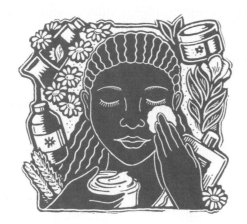

CHAPTER 5

CONTACT ALLERGIES AND SKIN REACTIONS

Disorders of the skin are among the most common problems that physicians have to deal with and conventional medicine has developed a battery of drugs to treat them. But this is one area where alternative remedies and therapies really come into their own. Natural strategies for controlling and managing skin problems can help to reduce the need for drugs or even make them unnecessary.

WHAT IS CONTACT ALLERGY?

Substances which cause an allergic reaction on contact with the skin are called contact allergens; the reaction that they cause is called contact allergy.

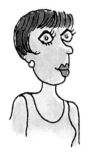

Brunettes have less vulnerable skin than blondes

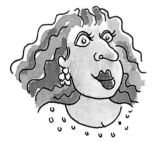

Redheads have the most vulnerable skin

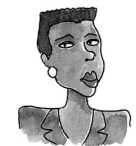

Black skin is probably the most resistant to irritants

Rashes may be caused in many ways – as symptoms of illnesses such as measles or streptococcal sore throat, as reactions to ingested or inhaled toxic substances, by contact with a toxin (for instance stinging nettles or irritant chemicals) or from nutritional deficiencies (such as deficiencies of B vitamins). Everyone may suffer from these, although some people's skin is more sensitive than others.

In addition, allergic individuals may develop rashes in reaction to a food or drug they have ingested (for instance penicillin) or even from allergens, such as mould, that they have inhaled. Allergic people can also develop contact reactions from substances which are harmless to other people. These include some plants and animals, house dust and house dust mites, elastoplast, nickel in jewellery, some fabrics or the finishes on new fabrics, foods and low concentrations of some chemicals.

People who continually have skin reactions become what is called 'hyper-reactive' and may even start to develop rashes from emotional scenes, or from exposure to sunlight or cold. If the sufferer can avoid the allergens most of the time this hypersensitivity may gradually lessen.

DIFFERENT TYPES OF SKIN ALLERGY

The range of terms used to describe types of skin allergy can be confusing. The main terms are urticaria, eczema and dermatitis.

Urticaria (also called nettle-rash or hives) is a very itchy rash associated with reddening of the skin and whitish bumps, usually small but sometimes as much as an inch or more across. The rash is short-lasting but may appear in a series of waves, going on for months. It affects the middle layers of the skin, but may also affect the lower layers, resulting in swelling which is called angio-oedema.

Eczema is a more chronic type of skin rash which develops more slowly and is usually less itchy. Atopic eczema is the term used for the condition in patients who have atopy – the general predisposition for developing allergic reactions, also involved in asthma, rhinitis, urticaria and Type A food allergy. Contact eczema is an allergic reaction provoked by contact, for instance, with jewellery or coins. However, the term eczema is also often used for rashes which are not known to be caused by an allergy, particularly in children.

Dermatitis is a wider term used to cover conditions due to irritation or to allergies, and is also used for some other skin conditions. Dermatitis is the term used for industrial skin diseases, many of which are said to be contact dermatitis. If the condition is clearly allergic in origin, it is called allergic contact dermatitis.

ALLERGY VERSUS IRRITATION

An irritant is a substance – such as solvent in paint – that breaks through the protective outer layers of the skin and causes damage and irritation. Irritants can cause dermatitis, which can make the skin more vulnerable to infection, or, in allergic individuals, sensitise the skin so that the irritant or another substance can produce an allergic reaction – allergic eczema.

Irritants are harmful to anyone's skin (although some people may be more sensitive than others). In contrast, contact allergens may be completely harmless to most individuals. Even in allergic people, their effects are likely to be delayed – anything from a few hours to two days – making it hard to identify what is acting as a trigger.

WHO IS SUSCEPTIBLE?

Eczema in an infant is one of the first signs of atopy, a generalised tendency to hypersensitivity which is partly genetic in origin. This means that a tendency to develop skin allergy may be inherited, and that children of allergic parents are more at risk. As with other allergic conditions, environmental factors in the early years of life are also important.

The state of your skin

Dry, broken, cut or abraded skin is far more susceptible to allergens and irritants. Disorders which produce some of these conditions therefore increase susceptibility to skin allergies. For instance, people with ichthyosis, where the skin is abnormally dry (about 10 per cent of the UK population), are very vulnerable, and their skin condition benefits if they take a holiday in the humidity of the tropics. Conversely, sweat can make the skin more vulnerable, as it dissolves and spreads some allergens – nickel from buttons for instance.

Other influences on the skin include excess sunlight, extremes of temperature and exposure to harsh weather. Any of these can chap the skin, damage its pH balance, dry it out and generally make it more vulnerable. The skin thins and weakens

HOW IRRITATION AND ALLERGY DIFFER

The distinctions between allergy and irritation reflect the different ways in which they cause damage to the skin – allergy only occurs when there is a hypersensitivity response.

	IRRITATION	ALLERGY
Cause of symptoms/ condition	Direct damage from irritant	Reaction to low concentrations of normally harmless substance
Who is vulnerable?	Everyone (although people's skins vary in toughness)	Minority of people who have been sensitised
Long-term effects	Skin may harden and become resistant, but most damage heals without lasting scars	Skin remains sensitive to very low concentrations of allergen. Allergic skin reactions may be chronic – lasting for a long time – or they may be recurrent

with age, which means that contact allergies are more common in older people (although skin reactions to other sources of allergen happen more in children and infants).

Nutrition and skin

Nutrition is a crucial factor in skin health. The lipid content of the top layer of the skin needs to be maintained at a healthy level. Deficiencies in diet or a poorly functioning metabolism can compromise this, but a diet rich in essential fatty acids (see page 108) can help to guard against skin problems, and there is evidence that evening primrose oil, which is rich in the EFA gamma-linolenic acid, can improve eczema.

THE SKIN'S DEFENCES

Skin is composed of two main layers – the epidermis, which provides the body's first line of defence against hostile organisms and substances, and the dermis. Lying underneath these is a layer of subcutaneous fat.

The epidermis has a top layer of dead cells filled with a protein called keratin, all set in a matrix of lipids (fats and oils). The keratin layer is the main defence against irritants, and can also withstand a lot of mechanical and chemical damage.

The dermis is composed mainly of dense but springy collagen, a protein that gives skin its elasticity and shock-absorbing capacity. Running through the dermis there are many blood vessels, which help with temperature regulation.

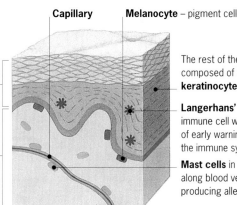

Capillary

Melanocyte – pigment cell

The rest of the epidermis is composed of live cells called **keratinocytes**.

Langerhans' cell, a type of immune cell which acts as a sort of early warning for the rest of the immune system.

Mast cells in the dermis and lying along blood vessels are important in producing allergic skin responses.

COMMON SYMPTOMS OF SKIN ALLERGIES

Itching, redness and swelling are common features of allergic skin reactions. Understanding the course of your condition is a vital first step towards coping with and treating such symptoms.

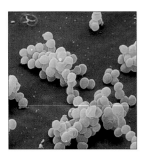

STAPHYLOCOCCUS AUREUS
This bacteria, seen here under a scanning electron microscope, is a common invader of broken skin, such as that produced by scratching. It can worsen inflammation and irritation.

SYMPTOMS AND LAYERS
Different symptoms and effects are produced in the skin according to which layer is affected.

Disorders of the top layer produce eczema (or dermatitis)

Disorders of the middle layer produce urticaria

If problems spread to the subcutaneous layer, severe swelling (angio-oedema) results

Skin reactions exhibit a set of common symptoms, as well as ones particular to the condition. Characteristic reactions include redness of the skin (erythema), accompanied by raised bumps (weals) and blisters (vesicles) of fluid, which may weep or ooze, or join up to give larger blisters. The skin may itch to various degrees; scratching the itch gives rise to a further set of consequences.

ECZEMA AND DERMATITIS

These are chronic conditions involving redness and inflammation of the skin, which tends to thicken and become rough and flaky. Severity varies – increased itchiness is often a sign that it is getting worse. The severity of the itching ranges from minimal to moderate, and occasionally severe. If the condition is acute, tiny bubbles or vesicles develop within the skin which may coalesce to form blisters which may burst and weep. Very chronic forms involve dryness of the skin and flaking on the surface that becomes steadily thicker until deep fissures form. These are painful and may bleed. Most commonly, intermediate forms between these two extremes are seen. The dermatitis heals without scarring or residual damage, even after a chronic course lasting for years.

More than one mechanism may be involved and any part of the body may be affected, from small to large areas. The hands are affected in 50 per cent of cases. If the whole body surface is involved, a condition known as erythroderma, this can have serious consequences for the well-being of the individual. Erythroderma can cause excessive heat loss, failure to regulate body temperature, dehydration and mineral depletion; it may lead to heart failure in the elderly.

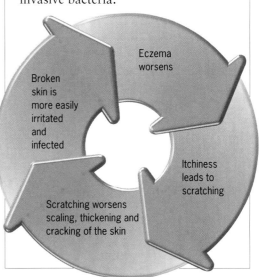

THE VICIOUS CYCLE OF SCRATCHING

Once the skin is broken it becomes more vulnerable to irritants and allergens, and may be infected with invasive bacteria.

Eczema worsens

Itchiness leads to scratching

Scratching worsens scaling, thickening and cracking of the skin

Broken skin is more easily irritated and infected

Childhood eczema

Mostly affecting children of allergic families this usually starts in the first year of life, sometimes within a few days of birth, and it often clears up by puberty. It may affect the face, body, limbs or nappy area and localise in the flexures (the insides of the elbows, knees, etc.) in the second year. Flexural eczema is often due to foods, most often milk and eggs, but children with eczema should not be put on elimination diets without medical supervision and precautions – there have been reports of serious reactions after challenges. Eczema on the outer side of the limbs is more likely to be due to contact with dust mite allergens or chemicals which may be found on carpets. Small children need to be allowed to crawl, however, so protect them with frequently washed long cotton trousers and long sleeved tops.

Eczema in adults

In adults, eczema is usually divided into exogenous eczema, meaning it is caused by something from outside the body, in other words by allergy or irritation – and idiopathic, which means of unknown origin. Some forms of eczema are regarded as non-allergic because no cause has been identified, although sometimes this may be because a number of triggers are involved so avoiding only one of them makes little difference. Others, such as hypostatic eczema in the elderly, are genuinely non-allergic.

ACNE COSMETICA

Sometimes adults of 20 or 30 upwards, suddenly develop spots and blemishes on their faces. Like contact eczema, the condition more commonly affects women because it is almost always due to cosmetics – as indicated by its name. The ingredients of many cosmetics can irritate the skin and cause allergic reactions. The simplest treatment is to stop using the cosmetics which cause the problem, but sufferers may have sensitive skin which needs special care.

URTICARIA

Commonly known as hives or nettle-rash, urticaria is often, but not always, caused by an allergic reaction. It can be caused by direct skin contact with either a toxin or an allergen, or by ingesting or inhaling one. For instance, urticaria is a classic consequence of allergic reaction to nuts or shellfish. An extremely itchy red rash appears on the skin and localised swellings develop, caused by the blood vessels leaking plasma (the watery part of the blood) into the surrounding tissue. These appear as raised white dots on a red background – the same effect as a mosquito bite, or indeed a nettle-rash – and are known as weals. If the swellings grow to a centimetre or more across the condition is called giant urticaria.

Angio-oedema

About 50 per cent of people with urticaria develop angio-oedema. This is characterised by swelling of deeper tissues. It particularly affects the lips, eyes and genital area. Angio-oedema can be serious if it affects the tongue or throat and medical help should be sought speedily.

Acute and chronic urticaria

Acute urticaria causes intense itching which comes on quickly and usually goes within 24 hours (but can last for a few days). It can be caused by foods, insect bites or stings, drugs like penicillin, or substances and materials in contact with the skin. It may be accompanied by collapse, nausea and fever, in which case the term anaphylaxis is more appropriate (see page 127). As the symptoms appear so rapidly, it can often be linked to an obvious cause, which should be avoided in the future.

Chronic urticaria is much more difficult to pin down and some sufferers never learn what triggers their condition. It can last for months or even years – not continually, but constantly appearing and then fading on different parts of the body. In some patients it is linked with food triggers, though not necessarily food allergy. Some foods (such as fish or sauerkraut) are naturally high in histamine, and in individuals who do not readily break down histamine this may trigger symptoms directly (this is not the same as an allergy). In other patients urticaria seems to be due to abnormal populations of organisms in the gut, such as fungi. For these patients a diet low in fermented foods, sugar and other refined carbohydrates, but with live yoghurt, is helpful.

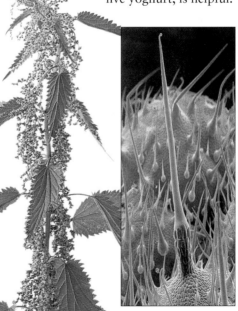

STINGING NETTLE
Urticaria is also known as nettle-rash because the stinging nettle, Urtica dioica, *causes the same reaction on contact with the skin. The surfaces of nettle leaves are covered with sharp, hollow hairs which contain histamine.*

COMMON ALLERGENS AND IRRITANTS

For anyone with vulnerable skin, it is important to be aware of the potential dangers posed by many cosmetics, cleaning products and other chemicals encountered in day-to-day life.

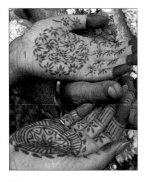

TRADITIONAL MAKE-UP
An Indian girl uses henna, a plant pigment, to trace designs on the palms of her hands– pigments made from both plants and minerals have been used for millennia.

OVERALL COVER
Some of the chemicals used in gardening may provoke a skin reaction, and gardeners may also need to protect themselves from the saps of grass and pine trees.

Human beings have been using make-up, wearing ornaments, piercing their bodies and working with metals for millennia, yet this century has seen a startling rise in the incidence of eczema, just as it has with rhinitis and asthma. It is entirely probable that prehistoric men and women suffered from skin irritation due to toxic pigments, metal ornaments and rough fabrics, but contact allergies are a relatively modern phenomenon. What has changed?

The cosmetics we use now include a huge number of artificial compounds. Equally, artificial and often highly potent chemicals are now in everyday use in a variety of domestic and occupational contexts.

Perhaps the most significant factor is the marked rise in allergies in general. The increasing incidence of contact eczema probably reflects this rise, which may itself be linked to our increasing exposure to artificial chemicals (see page 57).

PLANTS

The classical triggers of contact urticaria are nettles and poison ivy. These plants have defence mechanisms that cause an irritant skin reaction in anyone who touches them, but for some people the consequences can be severe, with widespread and lasting rash. Poison ivy (and poison oak) are more of a problem in America than Europe. The juices and saps in the stems of many plants can be irritants or allergens (some interact with sunlight to cause a reaction, a phenomenon known as phototoxic dermatitis), and many of the chemicals used in gardening can cause reactions, so wear gloves when handling them, and wear long sleeves and trousers when working in the garden.

WATER

Prolonged exposure to water can break down the protective lipid outer barrier of the epidermis and cause chapping. This makes the skin more vulnerable to further reactions. Use cotton-lined rubber gloves to protect your skin.

FACIAL COSMETICS

There are so many potential triggers in cosmetics that it is impossible to list them all. Common culprits are dyes, preservatives and fragrances that manufacturers add to most products – substances like benzyl salicylate, or phenylacetaldehyde.

OCCUPATIONAL EXPOSURE

Contact dermatitis is a serious problem for employers and workers alike. It is the most common occupational disorder – according to one estimate some 4 million working days are lost annually in the UK because of the complaint. It is mainly the hands that are affected, and some professions are more hazardous than others. Catering workers, hairdressers, mechanics and cleaners are all at risk because they have so much contact with detergents, solvents and water.

If one type of cosmetic causes a reaction, you can probably find another type with different ingredients that won't. Hypo-allergenic products may be better tolerated.

FOODS

Food allergies are a common cause of both acute and chronic skin problems. Foods cause problems both from ingestion and from contact. Some estimates blame more than half of childhood eczema on food allergy. The main food allergens are milk and eggs, but many other foods may be involved. Additives such as artificial colourings, flavourings and preservatives may also cause reactions.

RUBBER

Some of the ingredients of rubber, including latex, can cause allergies. Latex is used for disposable gloves, which are ubiquitous in the health industry and in many other situations involving the handling of hazardous substances (the powder used to lubricate the gloves can also cause problems). Alternative gloves are available but are more expensive. Latex condoms and diaphragms can also cause problems (see Chapter 7). Reactions to latex can range from mild eczema to full-blown anaphylaxis (see page 127).

SOAPS AND DETERGENTS

Detergents are designed to bond to fats and oils, allowing them to be washed away. As a result, prolonged exposure to detergents will also strip the skin of its protective fats and oils. Again, dish washers and cleaners are at particular risk.

Eczema sufferers should avoid using soap or use a mild, non-perfumed soap and follow baths and showers with emollients. Sensitive people may react to contaminants in tap water when washing – installing a filter with an activated carbon element in the water system or showerhead can help.

Some washing powders cause problems which may be due to the nature of the detergent or enzymes, or the perfumes. Using non-biological powders and careful rinsing (perhaps putting clothes through a second wash cycle without any powder) can help – most sufferers can find a washing powder they can tolerate. If not, clothes can be washed in sodium bicarbonate or borax (a common water softener and cleaning agent). Fabric conditioners should be avoided.

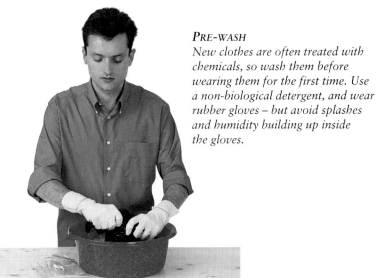

CLOTHING AND FABRICS

Allergy sufferers are often unable to tolerate new clothes until they have been washed. Wool and cotton can sometimes act as allergens, but in general it is artificial fibres that cause the most problems, especially polyester, viscose or rayon. Potential skin allergy sufferers should wear loose cotton clothing, and use pure cotton bedding; linen or silk are possible alternatives.

METALS

Nickel is a common cause of allergy, probably because of its widespread use in jewellery, especially earrings, and in coinage. The prevalence of ear piercing among women may explain why they are more likely to have contact reactions than men. According to a Danish study in 1994, some 11 per cent of Danish women are allergic to nickel. About half the young women who are allergic to nickel will later develop eczema, but can often tolerate pure gold (preferably 18-carat, for purity).

Other troublesome metals include chromium, which causes problems as an ingredient of cement (as chromate), and in leather goods, bleach and matches. Some intra-uterine devices are made from copper, which can cause problems for the women using them.

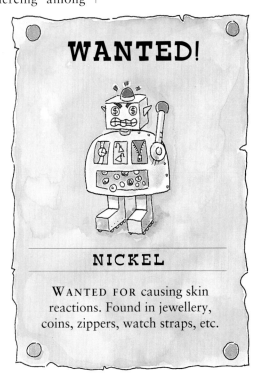

WANTED!

NICKEL

WANTED FOR causing skin reactions. Found in jewellery, coins, zippers, watch straps, etc.

Choosing Products That Are

Hypo-allergenic

There are many skincare, health and beauty products on the market which are labelled hypo-allergenic. Even bedspreads, detergents and clothing can be hypo-allergenic. So what exactly does the term mean?

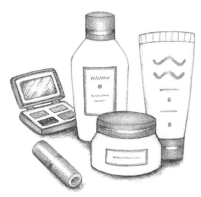

NOT PERFUMED, NOT COLOURED
Most pharmacies stock a range of products labelled as hypo-allergenic, but this may not mean much. The amount of information provided on the label can tell you how well researched the product is.

Taking care of your skin means being gentle with it, and using products that contain a minimum of irritants or potential allergens. At the same time you need to be able to clean yourself, your clothes and your home effectively, and use cosmetics, scents and deodorants if you choose. This is where hypo-allergenic products come in. Hypo-allergenic means 'with less potential to cause an allergic reaction' – in other words, low allergenicity. A hypo-allergenic product is one that, in theory, is specially formulated to fit this definition.

But how safe are hypo-allergenic products really? Are they all the same? And how do you know which ones to choose?

SOME FACTS ABOUT HYPO-ALLERGENICS

In practice 'hypo-allergenic' is a slightly nebulous term. There are no set guidelines or rules for manufacturers wishing to label their products as hypo-allergenic, other than the vague proviso that they must be less likely to cause an adverse reaction than comparable products. The degree to which each product avoids potential irritants and allergens differs widely. Some manufacturers simply leave out fragrances, the major source of problems, but leave in other well-known troublemakers like parabens.

People have different sensitivities and levels of reactivity, so one person might react to a product that another person would find safe. Finding the right product involves two steps: first, you need to check the ingredients and tests done on the product; and second, try testing some of the product on yourself. You can do this either with a DIY patch test (see page 110), or simply by rubbing a little on your inner forearm. Repeat this test twice daily for up to four days. You could also try a smell test – sometimes people who are hypersensitive to chemicals can tell simply by sniffing that a product or substance will cause them to have an adverse reaction.

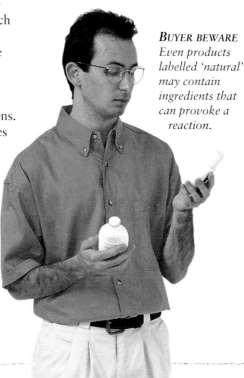

BUYER BEWARE
Even products labelled 'natural' may contain ingredients that can provoke a reaction.

WHAT TO LOOK FOR

▶ *Stick to reputable manufacturers.*

▶ *Get the information you need from the product label, or alternatively contact the manufacturer.*

▶ *Use this information to check which tests have been done on the product. Things to look for are tests for irritancy, sensitising potential, phototoxicity (whether it becomes more troublesome with exposure to sunlight), repeat insult patch tests, microbiological challenge tests and tests to check whether the product clogs pores (termed comedogenicity).*

▶ *Check for common trigger ingredients that may be irritant or allergenic – look out especially for preservative, benzocaine, alcohol, dyes and colourings (such as azo dyes), parabens and lanolin.*

▶ *Always remember to follow the instructions – for instance, storage at the wrong temperature may cause the contents to alter in some way and become irritant.*

TREATING SKIN ALLERGIES

Many creams, ointments and medications are available for treating skin reactions. However, side effects may be a problem, and alternative therapies have a great deal to offer.

Avoidance of the allergens or irritants is the best treatment for skin reactions. Some irritants and allergens are easy to avoid but in many cases the nature of the triggers is not clear. It is worth persisting, however, because even reducing your exposure to only a few triggers may make it much easier to control symptoms.

CONVENTIONAL TREATMENTS
In cases where there is no obvious cause, doctors are very likely to rely on medications, mainly creams and lotions, to control the problem. However, a problem which is often overlooked is that some patients react to one of the ingredients, exacerbating their conditions.

Emollients
An emollient is a substance that soothes and softens the skin. It is important for restoring the moisture and lipid content of the skin, helping to keep it flexible and making it less vulnerable to cracking, irritants and damage. There are many commercial varieties, but these may be expensive, or even contain irritating or allergenic ingredients. Using oil in a tepid bath (people with skin reactions should avoid excessive heat) can be a natural alternative: try olive or almond oil – as long as you're not allergic to them – or a few drops of some of the aromatherapy oils.

Calendula or elder and almond cream can be very soothing for itchy or weeping rashes. Apply calendula cream with caution at first in case it causes irritation.

Topical steroids
These are the main form of medication for eczema, and have an extremely good record – used in small amounts and kept away from the eyes these are safe. However, there is concern about the safety of heavy usage, because steroids can be absorbed through the skin. Atrophy of the skin is the most troublesome side effect: over time the skin can become thin, and irreversible disfigurement may result.

In severe cases the relief these medications provide outweighs the negative factors, but their regular use by patients with mild eczema is a different matter, especially if the patients have not attempted to find out the provoking factors. It is particularly important to relieve the itchiness of eczema, because the scratching that results initiates a damaging vicious cycle (see page 102). Non-drug treatments can help to relieve itching and reduce the need for steroids.

Other conventional treatments
Systemic steroids, given orally or as injections, are sometimes used in short courses to control an attack. In severe cases they may be needed regularly but this risks side effects in the long term, including osteoporosis and thinning of the skin. Ultraviolet light treatment, given in combination with a light-sensitive drug, is sometimes used to reduce the skin's tendency to produce an allergic response. Immuno-suppressive drugs, such as cyclosporin, can produce a rapid response in atopic eczema but can also cause kidney damage, hypertension and hair and gum problems, and improvement may only last as long as the treatment is taken.

Iatrogenic disease
Disease caused by the doctor's actions or prescriptions is termed iatrogenic, and iatrogenic disorders make up a serious proportion of skin reactions. According to some estimates, approximately one-third of all allergic contact dermatitis is iatrogenic.

EMOLLIENT OILS
Aromatherapy oils, such as camomile, lavender, juniper and geranium can be added to the bath for emollient effect.

DRUG-FREE ITCH RELIEF

The basic principles of drug-free relief from itching are keeping the skin cool and moist, and avoiding irritation. Simple measures include rubbing ice cubes on the skin, and applying cold, wet compresses. You can make these out of crushed ice cubes wrapped in wet cotton. Dressings like this help to cool inflammation, relieve itching and prevent oozing and weeping. Follow up cold compresses with calamine lotion or dressings of zinc oxide paste (available from pharmacists). Cool baths with added oil (such as olive or a few drops of aromatherapy oil), oatmeal, baking powder or corn starch can help to soothe and rehydrate the skin. A little vinegar in water can soothe and help to restore the correct pH balance of the skin (pH 6–7). Avoid using soap or use non-perfumed, mild soaps in the bath, and moisturise your skin afterwards with gentle, non-perfumed preparations. Other recommendations are to use cotton clothes and sheets, stay out of the sun, and stay cool. Also, try to keep a constant but moderate level of humidity in the house.

KEEP MOIST
Your skin can dry out after a bath, so use a non-fragranced moisturiser.

Cooling foods

In Chinese medicine cooling foods are recommended which nourish the yin and disperse the hot yang energy to reduce irritation. A naturopath may pursue the same effect by prescribing a raw food diet which excludes all sweet foods, even honey and dried fruits.

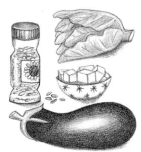

STAY COOL
Cooling foods include sunflower seeds, aubergine, lettuce and tofu.

NATURAL TREATMENTS

Effective natural alternatives are worth exploring. Relieving itchiness and preventing the negative cycle of scratching and damage is the first step, but do other treatments go deeper?

Evening primrose oil (EPO)

Deficiencies in the intake and processing of essential fatty acids (EFAs) have been linked to eczema (see page 101). Evening primrose oil is rich in EFA and has been shown to improve eczema. A 1982 study on 60 adults and 39 children, at the Bristol Royal Infirmary, England, showed improvement in itching after taking EPO for twelve weeks. EPO is available both over the counter and on prescription.

Chinese medicine

The herbal remedies that have been used for centuries in traditional Chinese medicine have sparked interest because of claims that they can cure severe, chronic atopic dermatitis where conventional medicine has failed. In practice the people who derive most benefit from Chinese medicine are patients who are not severely affected, but the same holds true for practically any medical treatment. Practitioners of Chinese medicine also prescribe remedies for the treatment of urticaria.

Chinese herbal remedies are usually taken as decoctions – infused in boiling water like a tea. These 'teas' may be extremely unpleasant to drink, and more palatable freeze-dried preparations of the complex mixtures are available on prescription. The remedies seem to be effective in about half of cases. However, the action of the herbs is not well understood, and there is known to be a risk of kidney or liver damage due to lack of control and regulation of potentially toxic ingredients. Any patient taking this treatment should be thoroughly monitored by a doctor.

Other alternative remedies

Opinions are divided over the benefits of homeopathy in eczema treatment, but there are several remedies commonly used for urticaria, including *Apis mellifica*, *Urtica urens* and *Dulcamara*. Naturopathy is an obvious option to try because food allergies are common triggers of both urticaria and dermatitis.

Herbal remedies can be useful – calendula, chickweed and aloe vera ointments can help with soreness, dryness and itching. Camomile lotion can help relieve the inflammation of urticaria. All of these herbal options should be used with caution in case you are allergic or sensitive to the plants or close relatives.

PREVENTING SKIN ALLERGIES

Prevention is always better than treatment, and treating skin allergies is often difficult. Taking care of your skin by following basic precautions can help you to stay healthier and happier.

Extreme conditions are the enemy of sensitive skin. Sweating can irritate the skin and block up the pores; dryness can crack it open and strip it of its protective properties. Heat can inflame (and cause sweating) while exposure to cold, windy weather can cause chapping. Prolonged immersion in water, astringent soaps and rough clothes will all damage, dry and chafe the skin.

AVOIDING EARLY EXPOSURE

When there is a strong family history of allergies, taking precautions during late pregnancy and during the first year of life reduces the incidence of eczema. Mothers should consider avoiding allergenic foods such as milk products, eggs, fish, nuts and any foods to which they themselves are sensitive, both during the last three months of pregnancy and during lactation. They should also consider not giving their infants unhydrolysed cow's milk or soya milk, eggs, fish, wheat or orange until over nine

months, and take steps to reduce exposure to house dust mites. It may help for the mother to take supplements of vitamins, minerals (using a product designed specially for pregnancy and lactation) and evening primrose oil, which is rich in essential fatty acids – young babies are more likely to have eczema if their mother's milk is low in essential fatty acids. Be careful too about exposing infants to chemicals and to other allergens such as pets and high pollen counts. In particular, you should keep your child's sensitive skin away from cosmetics – either yours or ones marketed at children.

TREATING YOUR SKIN GENTLY

The first rule of good skin care should be to treat your skin gently. Basic beauty and skin-care guidelines apply here. Both men and women with sensitive skin should follow much the same rules as apply to those seeking to avoid wrinkles.

Avoid overexposure to the sun and protect yourself from its damaging rays with sunscreens. Remember to take care when choosing a sun lotion: sunscreens may contain substances like benzocaine or cinnamon oil, or various fragrances which may provoke a reaction.

Never allow your skin to dry out – use mild, non-fragranced, hypo-allergenic moisturisers and emollients and try to reduce the number of baths and showers you take. Pat yourself dry after washing, rather than rubbing. Be particularly aware of the moisture content of your skin in dry climates (hot or cold), or in rooms with air conditioning.

Use simple cosmetics and body-care products to minimise the number of ingredients that come into contact with your skin (for example, hypo-allergenic products – see

---

WARNING

It is important to warn your doctor if you know that you have sensitive skin or are allergic to a drug or medication. His or her choice of treatment will be influenced by this information, because some oral or topical antibiotics and skin treatments are more likely to cause trouble than others. The doctor also needs to know if you are allergic to latex or a metal, especially if you need surgery.

BIOHAZARDS
Watch out for extreme conditions that can dry or chafe your skin.

Heat increases the severity of inflammation, and makes you sweat – itself an irritant.

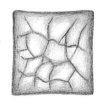

Dryness robs your skin of protective moisture, making it vulnerable to cracking.

Immersing your skin in water for long periods of time can strip it of protective oils.

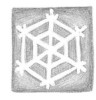

Extreme cold can cause chapping, especially in windy or wet conditions.

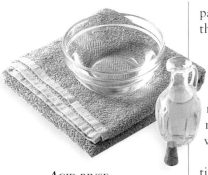

ACID RINSE
Adding a little vinegar to water (60 ml/2 fl oz in 1.2 litres/2 pints of water) can make a handy acidic treatment to maintain your skin's correct pH level.

page 106). Once you have found a cosmetic that works for you, stick with it – but be aware that as people get older they can develop allergies or intolerances to products they have used for years.

To protect your skin's pH level use mildly acidic soaps or apply special ointments (for instance those containing urea, which may sting), or try vinegar in water.

If you start to use a new product be cautious and keep an eye out for any warning signs or early symptoms of a reaction. The sooner you stop exposing your skin to an irritant or allergen, the less damage will be done and the easier it will be to recover. However, remember that if you do not react to it at first it does not prove that you will not become allergic or sensitive to that substance later on.

STRESS AND RELAXATION
The health of your skin is regarded as a key indicator of mental health, particularly for people with sensitive skin – in fact the skin has been described as the window on the body because of the way in which it shows telltale signs of illness and changes of emotion. Stress, depression and fatigue can cause or exacerbate skin reactions of all sorts – urticaria in particular is made worse by stress. Part of the stress response is a heightened awareness of irritations such as itchiness, so that stressed people may scratch more, worsening skin conditions.

However, a healthy mind can have a direct, positive influence on your immune system, on the levels in your blood of inflammatory substances like histamine and anti-inflammatory substances like prostaglandins and on your general ability to fight back against disease.

The most effective step you can take towards controlling and minimising your urticaria or dermatitis, after finding and avoiding the triggers, may be to reduce the level of stress in your life and to learn to cope with stress more effectively.

> **WARNING**
> *Never do a self-test with any strong or concentrated chemical, and never apply a test substance to skin which is inflamed, sore or cracked.*

SELF-ADMINISTERING A PATCH TEST

If you have an unexplained skin reaction, or if you know that you have sensitive skin and are worried about the possible effect of a newly encountered substance, you can try a patch test to check. You should allow 48 hours for the test.

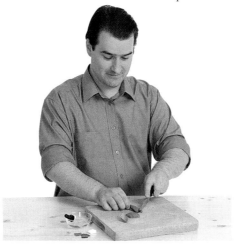

1 *Use a hypo-allergenic dressing to hold a sample of the substance – a piece of cloth, a leaf fragment, or a household substance at the concentration it would be in contact with your skin – in place on your forearm.*

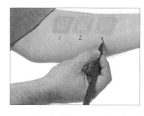

2 *Use a pen to code each substance on your skin (after checking that the ink does not produce a reaction). If a test site begins to itch, take the plaster off and consider the test positive.*

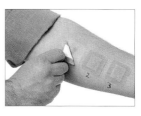

3 *Remove the plasters after 48 hours, wait for an hour, as the skin may be corrugated with moisture, and then look and feel for raised or red skin. Check again one and two days afterwards. If positive, avoid contact with that substance.*

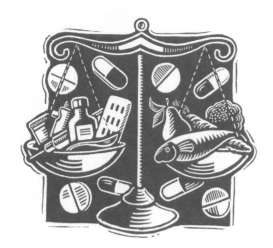

CHAPTER 6

DRUG ALLERGIES

The development of thousands of new drugs, and the increasingly widespread use of antibiotics, have led to a dramatic upsurge in the incidence of allergic reactions to drugs. But there are many ways to avoid the problems of drug allergy, and in learning to manage your allergy, you could also make dramatic improvements to your health.

ALLERGIES AND OTHER SIDE EFFECTS

Many drugs have unwanted side effects, but in sensitive individuals some drugs – including some of the most commonly used ones – can produce a potentially serious allergic reaction.

The role of a drug is, of course, to relieve symptoms and alter the course of an illness. Ideally the drug will work in a beneficial way – if it is an antibiotic it should work in tandem with the immune system to help it fight an invader. But drugs can also have a number of adverse effects. Where an adverse effect is produced by the immune reaction to the drug, it is said to be an allergic side effect.

SIDE EFFECTS

Effects produced by the drug which are neither intended nor therapeutic are said to be side effects. For instance, some antibiotics cause diarrhoea. This does not help them to work and is an unintended side effect which will vary in severity from patient to patient. There are three main types of side effect.

Pharmacological side effects

Pharmacological side effects are those which are produced by the direct action of the drug on the body, giving unwanted results. The desired effects of the drug are themselves pharmacological – the difference is simply between effects which are wanted and those which are unwanted.

Toxic side effects

The difference between a therapeutic effect and a toxic one is often just a matter of degree – of the size of the dose taken – and tolerances can vary from person to person. At a toxic dose, a drug is damaging rather than therapeutic. Licensing authorities usually demand a large safety margin between the prescribed dose and the lowest dose that is likely to cause serious harm.

Allergic side effects

Allergic side effects occur when the drug taker's immune system reacts to the drug, and an allergic response follows. This response may result in a variety of symptoms from rashes to full-blown anaphylaxis.

LEVELS OF SUSCEPTIBILITY

People differ in their susceptibility to the unwanted pharmacological effects of drugs, and to their toxic effects. For instance, some elderly people cannot tolerate doses of drugs which would be safe for most people. People deficient in some nutrients are also more susceptible to harmful effects caused by normally safe doses of drugs.

At the most extreme end of the spectrum, allergic individuals may suffer side effects from tiny amounts of a drug – doses far lower than those which would be toxic to non-allergy sufferers.

TOXIN TOLERANCE

Rasputin, a mysterious figure at the court of Tsar Nicholas II of Russia, is an extraordinary example of how people's tolerance for toxins can vary considerably. He was assassinated by Russian aristocrats worried by his influence at court, and during the ordeal he survived drinking enough cyanide to kill several men. He was finally drowned in the icy River Neva. His heavy drinking habits may have contributed to his unusual resistance to the cyanide.

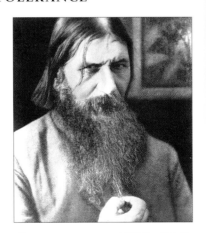

GRIGORY RASPUTIN (1871-1916)
Confidant of the Russian Tsarina, Rasputin was incredibly resistant to the toxic effects of cyanide.

SYMPTOMS OF DRUG ALLERGIES

Drug allergies are of serious concern to physicians, who need to be alert to the telltale signs of danger so that they can protect their patients and find effective alternative treatments.

There are a number of symptoms classically associated with drug allergy, but unfortunately they cannot be used as an infallible guide. Individually, each symptom can be caused by different conditions. On the other hand, symptoms can easily be misdiagnosed as something else, when the problem is indeed an allergy. Doctors need to use a blend of experience and careful scrutiny of the patient's history to determine whether allergies are to blame.

SKIN RASHES

The typical allergic rash is urticaria, otherwise known as hives or nettle rash. It manifests itself as very itchy white bumps, usually surrounded by red areas. Rashes can appear anywhere on the body.

Sometimes the bumps are large and join up to give giant urticaria, and the rash is often accompanied by areas of swelling, usually around the mouth, eyes and neck, known as angio-oedema. Some rashes take the form of dermatitis (see Chapter 5).

Not all rashes are allergic. In particular those associated with bleeding into the skin (which may appear as small red dots, not obvious to the non-specialist) are not usually allergic in nature.

> ### WARNING
> *Urticaria and angio-oedema can be followed by more severe allergic reactions if the same drug is taken again. Angio-oedema can also become dangerous if the throat swells up. See your doctor immediately if you notice sudden swelling of your tongue or throat.*

NAUSEA AND BOWEL PROBLEMS

Dizziness and blurred vision can cause nausea, but these are rarely caused by allergic reactions. Nausea is more commonly associated with allergic bowel disturbances, which also cause diarrhoea. Although such reactions are common, they are rarely recognised by doctors as being allergic in nature. Constipation can occur as an allergic effect, but is more often a non-allergic side effect, caused, for example, by preparations of iron given to combat anaemia or peptic ulcers.

HEADACHES AND FATIGUE

Vague and generalised reactions such as lethargy, fatigue and headaches are all common responses to drugs and may often be allergic in nature. They can be caused by minute quantities of the drug. However, these symptoms tend to be under-reported, and are often dismissed by doctors.

PHOTOSENSITIVITY

Allergy to drugs can make the skin sensitive to sunlight – bright sunlight will cause it to become red and sore, like an exaggerated sunburn. The condition sometimes persists for decades, and may be extremely disabling. Sufferers have to cover up, wear sunblock (which may provoke an irritant or allergic reaction in some people) and stay out of the sun. Long term exposure to tetracyclines, used to control teenage acne, can cause this condition.

ANAPHYLAXIS

Allergy to penicillin is one of the leading causes of anaphylaxis, although considering how many people take penicillin, it is a rare side effect. Injections are more likely to cause anaphylaxis than drugs taken orally.

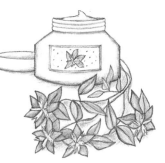

CHICKWEED OINTMENT
Herbalists recommend chickweed ointment for natural relief from the itchiness of urticaria.

COVER UP
Photosensitive people have to cover up, wear hypo-allergenic sunblock and stay out of the sun.

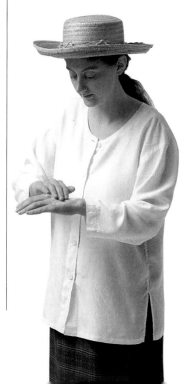

Common problem drugs

Most drug allergies are caused by a few commonly used drugs. Antibiotics are the main culprits, but anything from aspirin to vaccines can cause an allergic reaction.

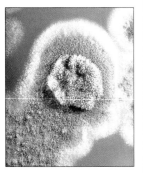

PENICILLIUM MOULD
Commonly found throughout the house, this mould naturally produces penicillin, and can cause allergies itself.

With any form of medication, a doctor weighs up the potential risks and benefits before prescribing it. This means that drugs which are known to be allergic troublemakers are still in common use because they are such powerful elements of the doctor's armoury. Most important of all are the antibiotics, which account for one in ten of GP prescriptions in the UK. Penicillins, a major class of antibiotics, are the most widely prescribed drugs in the world.

ANTIBIOTICS

The discovery of the antibacterial properties of penicillin earlier this century is a familiar tale, but antibiotics have been in use for thousands of years. The Chinese have been using mouldy soya bean curd as a locally applied antibiotic for at least two and a half millennia, while a traditional folkloric British treatment for cuts is an old cobweb. In all these cases the antibiotic effect derives from mould – or rather from substances that are produced by mould.

Penicillins

Of all the antibiotics, penicillins are the most common cause of drug allergies. A study in Boston in 1976 estimated that at least five per cent of the US population are allergic to the ampicillin form of penicillin. Typically, penicillin allergy causes a rash with itching, but in extreme cases it can trigger anaphylaxis, particularly if the patient has previously had a reaction.

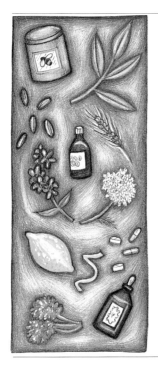

ANTIBIOTICS AND ALTERNATIVE REMEDIES

The table below shows the antibiotics that would most often be prescribed for a few common conditions, together with some other remedies that you could try.
Remember not to disregard your doctor's advice – this list is only a guide.

CONDITION	ANTIBIOTICS	OTHER TREATMENTS
Sore throat	Penicillins (narrow spectrum) Sulphonamides	Honey and lemon drink; gargle with salt water; inhale steam with olbas oil and Friar's balsam; red sage (*Salvia officinalis*) infusion – gargle every 4 hours; aspirin gargles (for adults)
Chest infections	Penicillins (broad spectrum)	Honey and lemon drink; warm liniment rub on back, chest and throat; hot infusion of elderflower, hyssop and white horehound; inhalation of warming aromatic oils such as eucalyptus; cough linctus
Ear infections	Penicillins Pain relievers (only with antibiotics)	Almond oil drops at body temperature; cotton wool compresses soaked in yarrow infusion and placed around ear; acupressure to relieve symptoms; hot compress on ear to soothe aches
Urinary infections	Tetracyclines Sulphonamides	Barley water – simmer barley and lemon peel, then add honey to the infusion; drink plenty of water and sodium bicarbonate; parsley tea; juniper berry, eucalyptus and sandalwood oil in a warm bath; cranberry juice as a preventative measure (but not a cure)

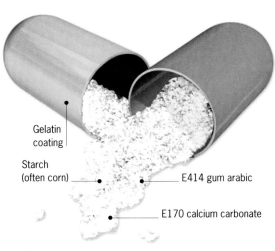

Gelatin coating

Starch (often corn)

E414 gum arabic

E170 calcium carbonate

ADDITIVES IN PILLS
Pills and capsules are mostly composed of substances like sugar or corn starch, known as excipients, which are used to carry the active ingredients. Many pills are coloured with additives such as azo-dyes, or flavoured with sugar coatings. Any of these excipients can cause an allergic reaction in a susceptible individual.

If any sort of reaction occurs, the patient should stop taking the drug immediately and the doctor will consider prescribing an alternative. If the trigger is subsequently avoided sensitivity may fade, but you should not resume taking a drug until instructed to do so, or, for serious reactions, until it has been shown by means of skin or blood tests conducted in a proper medical setting that you are not sensitive.

Other antibiotics

Some people who are allergic to penicillin may also be allergic to other antibiotics, especially the cephalosporins. Several other types of antibiotic can, albeit rarely, cause allergy in their own right. Macrolides, which include erythromycin and others, can cause gastric upsets which are not allergic, but can also cause true allergic reactions. Tetracyclines do not usually cause acute reactions but extended use as a treatment for acne may cause the build-up of derivative compounds. These are normally inert but can become transformed by sunlight into substances that provoke a reaction known as photodermatitis, in which bright sunlight causes an acute nettle rash (see photosensitivity, page 113).

Antibacterials

These are drugs which have similar uses to antibiotics, but are derived from chemical synthesis rather than from moulds and fungi. In particular, a common group of sulphur-based drugs, the sulphonamides, can cause rashes and other symptoms.

Antibiotics in food

Adding antibiotics and antibacterial agents to animal feed is a widespread practice in the agricultural industry. They are given to livestock, poultry and fish, and trace amounts can be found in meat, milk and eggs, though to what levels is unclear. Allergy sufferers are sensitive to even minute quantities of their trigger allergen, and there have been cases of reactions which seem to be due to antibiotic contamination of food.

ASPIRIN

Unlike antibiotics, pain-relieving drugs can be bought over the counter, and thus can be taken without any form of medical supervision. In some ways this makes them riskier than antibiotics – aspirin is the second most likely drug after penicillin to cause allergic reactions. Typical symptoms are itchiness and rash, and aspirin may also cause asthma and nasal polyps (small nodules in the nose or sinuses).

Aspirin, or salicylic acid, is derived from the bark of the willow tree (genus *Salix*). Some other plants contain related compounds called salicylates, and anyone who is allergic to aspirin should seek advice from a dietitian on avoiding foods with a high salicylate content, such as spices, peppers and apricots.

VACCINES

In the past vaccines were either made from horse serum or were cultured in eggs. This obviously posed problems for people allergic to horses or eggs. However, the amount of such material in modern treatments is very small, and current varieties of vaccine very rarely cause trouble. If you are sensitive to horses or eggs, however, always warn the practitioner before you are given a vaccination. If necessary, inoculations can always be given in hospital to be on the safe side.

THREE REASONS TO AVOID ANTIBIOTICS

Antibiotics are valuable in the fight against infection, but many doctors are growing more cautious in using them.

▶ *Over-prescription of antibiotics is leading to the evolution of drug-resistant strains of bacteria. Prescribing fewer drugs may help to slow this development.*

▶ *If your immune system is left to cope with minor infections on its own, you tend to develop stronger immunity so if the infection recurs you will be more able to fight it off, unaided by medication.*

▶ *Antibiotics may kill off some of the friendly bacteria in your gut. This makes it easier for unfriendly microbes to invade the gut, causing problems like diarrhoea.*

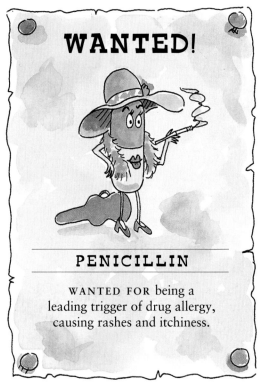

WANTED!

PENICILLIN

WANTED FOR being a leading trigger of drug allergy, causing rashes and itchiness.

The Acupuncturist

Acupuncture is an ancient Chinese treatment for illness which involves the insertion and manipulation of needles at carefully selected places in the body. It is an effective method of pain relief and, in China, is sometimes used as a surgical anaesthetic.

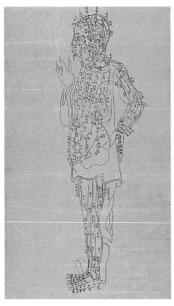

POWER LINES
This ancient Chinese illustration shows just a few of the major acupuncture points, part of a body of lore built up over thousands of years.

Acupuncture can help allergy sufferers in two ways. Firstly, it can be used to treat or relieve allergic symptoms directly, both acute allergic symptoms such as asthma, eczema and urticaria, and chronic Type B symptoms, like depression.

Secondly, acupuncture can help to reduce reliance on painkillers and other drugs – indeed in the West, acupuncture is mainly used for pain relief. This includes pain from injury, arthritis, nervous tension, PMS and dysmenorrhea (painful periods), migraine and sciatica. By acting as a side effect-free replacement for pain killers, acupuncture can reduce a

sufferer's need for medication, and therefore the risk of adverse reactions to drugs.

How does it work?

Acupuncturists believe that energy passes through channels (known as meridians) in the body, and that this energy can be accessed through carefully mapped points on the skin. Different meridians relate to different organs, so the insertion and manipulation of needles at the relevant points can relieve symptoms from these organs, as well as in other, seemingly unrelated parts of the body. Acupressure involves applying pressure to these points to achieve similar ends.

Acupuncture and acupressure points are found along the meridians, and are labelled according to their position. For instance, point KID 27 is the 27th point on the kidney meridian.

What qualifications and training will an acupuncturist have?

Some will have trained in China – courses approved by the Chinese are probably the best and certainly the hardest. However, in the West it can be difficult to verify claims about Eastern training, so it is generally wiser to use practitioners registered with one of the UK training bodies.

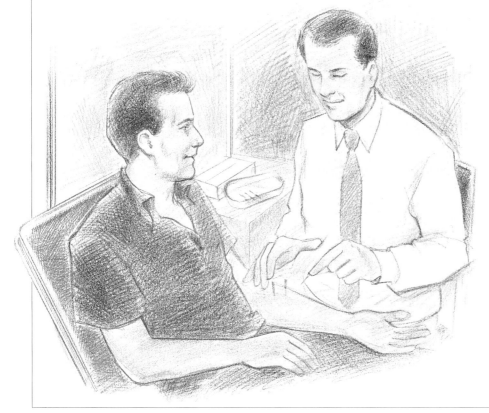

RELIEF POINTS
Acupuncture can provide direct relief from allergic symptoms, and can also reduce the need for analgesic drugs, lowering the chance of allergic reactions.

There are two main organisations in this country. The British Academy of Western Acupuncture organises short training programmes mainly intended for qualified doctors. Successful candidates become registered members and must adhere to a strict ethical code.

The new British Acupuncture Council registers practitioners who have trained and qualified as acupuncturists, either through a full-time course or on a postgraduate course following a healthcare qualification – such as a degree in osteopathy. It also has a register of members – there are more than 1000 practitioners – and an ethical code.

What evidence is there that acupuncture works?

Some proponents of acupuncture, including the British Academy of Western Acupuncture, believe that acupuncture cannot be assessed by normal scientific methods, and use anecdotal evidence to support their claims. The British Acupuncture Council, on the other hand, does support the use of controlled scientific investigations, while recognising the value of other approaches to testing.

Acupuncturists in other countries have not been so slow off the mark. A 1995 study at the Christian Albrechts University in Germany showed that acupuncture provided significantly more relief from migraine than a placebo treatment. A study of 192 patients published in the *Journal of Traditional Chinese Medicine* in 1990 showed that acupuncture could bring immediate relief to asthma sufferers, and was particularly effective for patients with a history of drug allergy. A controlled study in 1996, at the University Clinic of Physical Therapy and Rehabilitation, in the USA, showed that acupuncture on the ear could significantly increase the pain threshold of sixty volunteers. These are just three of a host of studies supporting the use of acupuncture for both pain relief and allergies.

ACUPRESSURE FOR ALLERGIC RHINITIS

Acupressure works on similar lines to acupuncture but uses finger pressure rather than needles to stimulate pressure points, and can be done anywhere. Acupuncturists recommend placing pressure for 2 minutes on the following points to relieve the itchy and runny eyes, sinuses and nasal passages of allergic rhinitis.

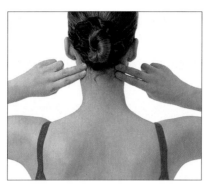

PRESSURE POINT BL 10
This is situated on either side of your spine, about two finger-widths below the base of your skull.

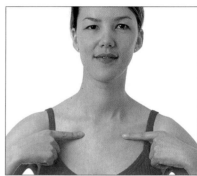

PRESSURE POINT KID 27
This is located just under your collarbones on either side of the breastbone.

What do conventional doctors think of it?

There is a wide spectrum of opinion, ranging from those who reject any medical application for acupuncture, to others who firmly believe in its value, in some cases using it regularly in addition to their conventional treatment methods.

Most doctors lie between these two extremes, and are happy for patients to use acupuncture in addition to other treatments. Indeed, among alternative treatments it is one of the most widely accepted, and when performed with proper precautions by a trained practitioner it is a very safe therapy. Virtually the only risk comes from transfer of infection from inadequately sterilised needles, and most acupuncturists now use disposable needles.

Who can and cannot benefit from acupuncture?

Skilled practitioners claim that there are few limitations to the range of conditions they can treat using acupuncture, but like any other form of therapy it will never be universally successful.

WHAT YOU CAN DO AT HOME

Acupuncture is strictly a specialist activity – one that you cannot perform yourself. Acupressure techniques, however, can be done at home to provide instant relief. Special bands with magnetised pellets are available which can help to apply constant electromagnetic stimulation to specific points. Your acupuncturist can advise if this is appropriate, recommend which points to focus on and show you how to use acupressure techniques.

PRESSURE BANDS
These bands press magnetised pellets against acupressure points, stimulating points on the ankles, wrists and arms.

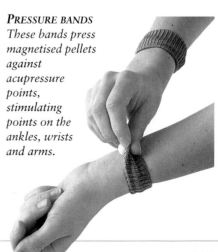

DRUGS AND NATURAL ALTERNATIVES

Natural remedies seem to provoke fewer allergic reactions than synthetic or highly processed drugs, but the only sure way of avoiding a reaction is to reduce your need for medication.

WEIGHING YOUR NEED FOR DRUGS
A decision to use medication is based on an assessment of the benefits it might provide versus the risk it entails. Doctors and patients alike must weigh up their options before deciding.

There are three cornerstones to reducing the likelihood of developing an allergic reaction to drugs. First, reassess your need for medication: do you really need to pop a pill, or will your complaint subside soon of its own accord? Second, substitute a simpler, natural remedy for a synthetic drug. Third, and most important, reduce your need for medication by improving your mental and physical well-being, so that you don't need to take any drugs in the first place.

RESTRICT YOUR DRUG USE

Any decision to take drugs should be based on necessity rather than convenience. Before reaching for the aspirin, ask yourself a few questions: do you have a serious problem, or simply a passing irritation? Is your problem self-limiting – in other words will it go away on its own without intervention? Can you effectively ignore it and get on with other activities? Are your symptoms telling you something you should not ignore? For instance, persistent headaches might indicate that you should look for the underlying cause, rather than using drugs.

Obviously there is a scale of severity. At one extreme, no one would seek to deny pain-relieving drugs to cancer sufferers, but at the other end of the scale, many people are guilty of over-reliance on painkillers and other drugs to cope with minor discomforts. Learn to weigh your need for medication against the possible risks and side effects it may produce.

BASIC PRECAUTIONS WITH DRUGS

Never self-medicate with prescription drugs or give medications specifically prescribed for you to others. Diagnosis is difficult enough even with the proper medical training. If you attempt to self-diagnose you risk missing important clues and misdiagnosing a severe or dangerous disorder. Self-medicating then compounds the mistake. Not only do you risk taking the wrong drug, but there may well be many subtleties of which you are not aware. Issues like the timing of doses and the dangers of interactions with other drugs means that the prescription of drugs requires expert training.

Minimise your use of drugs. Generally drugs should be a last, and not a first, resort. Try to get fit and healthy to prevent illness, and look for other ways of controlling simple problems.

Always follow instructions. The precise timing of your dose may be crucial: some must only be taken with food, or they will not be properly absorbed – for others the

DRUGS DON'T AGE WELL

Never use drugs after the expiry date shown on the label. The substances which make up a drug may be volatile or reactive, and their effectiveness depends on their exact composition. Like all substances – particularly organic ones, of which most pharmaceuticals are composed – they will degrade and break down with time. Some will merely become inactive, but others – such as the topical antibiotic tetracycline, often prescribed for sufferers of dermatitis – will actually become toxic with age. This applies to both prescription and over-the-counter medicines.

Stress Relief

Your state of mind can have an enormous influence on your physical health, including the strength of your immune system, your threshold for pain and your sensitivity to allergens. Reducing your stress levels can improve your mental health.

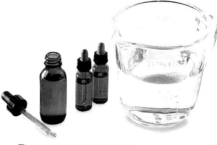

In order to control the stress in your life, and improve your health as a result, there are a number of lifestyle factors that you need to look at.

Planning

By allocating your time, learning to delegate and being prepared you can achieve your goals in the time allowed. Make a projected plan for the week ahead, and then keep a diary of what you achieve. Compare the two and identify what went right and where problems arose.

Exercise

Exercise can both relieve stress and make you more resistant to illness. Activities like t'ai chi can help you to get fit and teach you relaxation skills. You can even use stretching and flexibility exercises to combat pain directly, without drugs.

Natural stress relief remedies

Bach flower remedies are a safe means of counteracting stress and will not interfere with any medication you are taking.

CONCOCT YOUR OWN
Make your own Bach flower treatment mixture for stressful situations by diluting and mixing 2 drops each of any of the remedies below, in a 30 ml dropper bottle filled with mineral water.

Elm is a good remedy to use when feeling overwhelmed or unable to cope. Vervain helps to maintain energy levels, and soothes frustration. Impatiens can help when you feel that you can't keep up with a hectic schedule.

STRETCHES TO EASE TENSION

Stress and backache often go together, particularly in the office. Try the simple move shown here to help relieve tension and backache. Do not try this if you have severe back, muscle or joint problems – see a doctor, osteopath or physiotherapist.

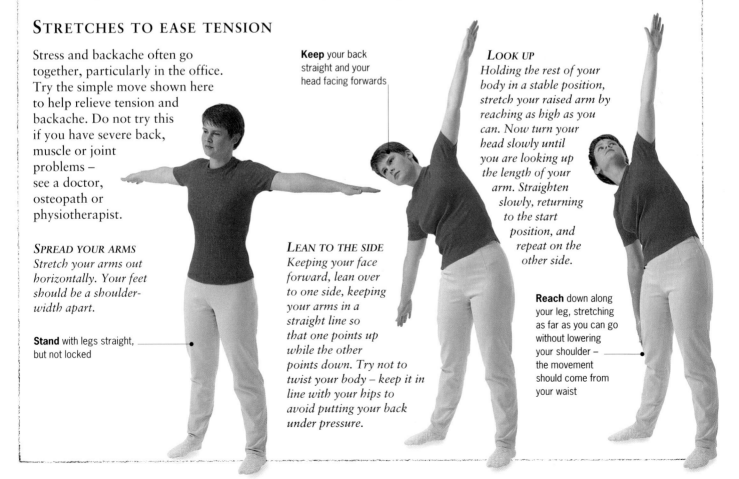

Keep your back straight and your head facing forwards

LOOK UP
Holding the rest of your body in a stable position, stretch your raised arm by reaching as high as you can. Now turn your head slowly until you are looking up the length of your arm. Straighten slowly, returning to the start position, and repeat on the other side.

SPREAD YOUR ARMS
Stretch your arms out horizontally. Your feet should be a shoulder-width apart.

Stand with legs straight, but not locked

LEAN TO THE SIDE
Keeping your face forward, lean over to one side, keeping your arms in a straight line so that one points up while the other points down. Try not to twist your body – keep it in line with your hips to avoid putting your back under pressure.

Reach down along your leg, stretching as far as you can go without lowering your shoulder – the movement should come from your waist

CLEAN LIVING
A healthy lifestyle, with exercise, good diet and low stress, is the best protection against ill health of all kinds, allergies included.

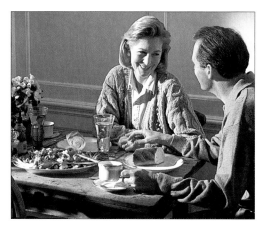

MEDICINE MAN
Shamans, witch doctors and medicine men, like the one below, rely overwhelmingly on natural remedies. Although these may provoke fewer allergic reactions than Western drugs, there are no safeguards against the inclusion of toxic ingredients – each side has its disadvantages.

opposite may be true. Some drugs must be taken regularly to maintain a therapeutic concentration in your bloodstream. Not following instructions can be dangerous.

NATURAL REMEDIES

The availability of drugs for managing pain, infections and other health problems is a relatively recent phenomenon. For most of our history we have relied on the sort of techniques that the majority of the world's population still relies upon – natural remedies prepared mainly from plants. These remedies often depend on potent active ingredients much the same as our modern pharmaceuticals, many of which are derived or developed from plant sources themselves.

This means that natural remedies should be approached with as much caution as conventional medicines – in some cases with more, because they may not have been properly tested and their manufacture is not regulated to such consistent standards.

Natural remedies can produce allergic reactions, but in general they are milder than conventional medicines and are probably less likely to cause problems. Homeopathic remedies in particular are generally very safe, since they involve the use of very low concentrations of substances (see Chapter 2). Nonetheless, you should always consult a qualified, registered herbalist, homeopath or other practitioner before using any natural remedies.

A HEALTHY LIFESTYLE

The best way to avoid using drugs is not to need them. The vast majority of minor complaints, and many of the major ones, are eminently preventable. A healthy, balanced diet, adequate exercise, moderate drinking,

not smoking, and reducing your stress levels make up the most effective preventative treatment you can find anywhere.

Poor diet and nutritional deficiencies are implicated in many allergic conditions, such as magnesium deficiency in asthma (see page 74), and in general physical and mental health. Lack of exercise can make you unfit and overweight – major risk factors for many types of disease. Exercise is an excellent way of reducing stress.

Alcohol and smoking are also implicated in many allergic illnesses and related conditions, both directly and indirectly. Alcohol and some of the elements of cigarette smoke can act as allergens or irritants themselves, exacerbating or causing allergic conditions such as asthma. Indirectly, they can impair general health and the functioning of the immune system.

Although allergic individuals will need to identify and avoid the substances that trigger their symptoms, the benefits of a healthy lifestyle could make a radical difference to the frequency and severity of these health problems. In fact by following a healthy lifestyle you can reduce the incidence in your life of headaches, migraine, sprains, aches, colds, stomach upsets, flu and infections of all kinds.

NATURAL REMEDIES FOR PAIN RELIEF

By cutting down on your use of drugs you can reduce the chances of developing an allergic reaction. One way of doing this is to treat mild illnesses with natural remedies.

Camphor oil and camomile tea may help to ease rheumatic pain. A poultice of feverfew is said to soothe migraine, and herbalists recommend gargling with red sage tea for relief from throat pain. Mint tea contains peppermint oil which may help with indigestion.

Hydrotherapy can be a simple and effective home remedy for many types of pain. Hot and cold compresses applied alternately for 20–30 minutes (3 minutes hot, 1 minute cold) may help to relieve many muscular and joint pains. The pain of a sore throat can be relieved with a cold compress.

CHAPTER 7

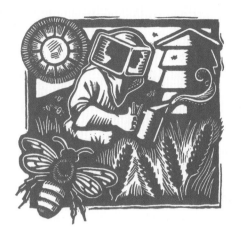

OTHER ALLERGIES

Inhalant, food, drug and contact allergies account for the vast majority of allergic reactions but there are many others. Some of them may afflict only a handful of people across the country, but this makes them no less serious: in very rare cases these conditions can cause fatal anaphylaxis.

Insect allergies

It is well known that wasp and bee stings can cause nasty reactions, even fatal anaphylaxis. In some cases other insects have also caused anaphylaxis, but such severe reactions are rare.

Fear of flying things
Only an unlucky few are in serious danger from an insect sting, and thanks to the treatment available, stings cause very few deaths each year. In the US, for instance, one person in six million dies from an insect sting per annum. In the UK the figure is nearer one in eleven million.

If you are going abroad and you know that you are allergic to wasp or bee stings, you should carry your own adrenaline kit (see page 128) at all times, together with a letter signed by your doctor explaining why you need it.

Reactions to insect bites and stings can take several forms. Most people suffer a local reaction after being stung, for instance by a wasp. The sting causes a small, inflamed swelling accompanied by a hot, throbbing pain – these symptoms generally clear up within a couple of days.

Someone is said to be allergic when a bite or sting produces an inappropriately severe reaction. In an allergic person the immune system overreacts, causing the release of histamine and other inflammatory agents. If this happens locally it gives a large swelling – a large local allergic reaction. If swellings appear at sites other than the actual sting, it is known as a systemic reaction – these can be very dangerous, and can even cause the fatal reaction known as anaphylactic shock.

Deaths from anaphylaxis caused by insect stings are extremely rare. Their annual incidence is about 40 in the US, 10 in Germany and 5 in the UK. That the death rate is this low is mainly due to patients taking precautions by carrying adrenaline and getting prompt medical attention, which is essential in any kind of systemic reaction – even if you think the danger has passed, you should still be checked by a doctor.

INSECTS THAT CAUSE ALLERGIES

Insects from the Hymenoptera group are the main cause of sting allergies, and the stings of these insects can produce serious reactions. The bee is potentially the most dangerous because it leaves its stinger in the skin of the victim, and the venom sac continues to pump poison. However, since most bees are not very aggressive, stings are quite rare. In practice, wasp and hornet stings are much more common due to their more aggressive nature and their habits. For instance, wasps are attracted to sweet foods and are thus drawn to eating places, where people are more likely to be stung.

LOCAL AND SYSTEMIC REACTIONS

In someone who is not allergic, the bite or venom causes localised reactions with a swelling of no more than 2 centimetres in diameter. In population surveys in the UK between 3 and 17 per cent of sting victims are reported to develop large local reactions – swellings of at least 10 centimetres in diameter which often last for more than 24 hours. Between 0.15 and 3.3 per cent of victims suffer a 'systemic' reaction.

Systemic reactions

A systemic reaction is a fairly immediate, generalised reaction which occurs in response to a sting. Anaphylaxis is actually the technical term for all systemic reactions, but it is usually used to mean a very severe reaction. Mild systemic reactions are characterised by itchy skin, swollen eyes and

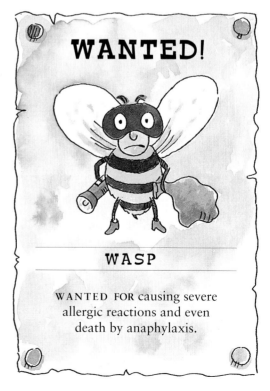

WANTED!

WASP

WANTED FOR causing severe allergic reactions and even death by anaphylaxis.

ALLERGENIC INSECTS

The insect group that causes the most allergy problems is the Hymenoptera. There are three insect families in this group: the Apidae (colloquially called the 'Apids') – honey bees and bumble bees; the Vespidae (the 'Vespids') – wasps and hornets; and the Formicidae, which includes the fire ant. Other insects whose bite or sting have been known to cause allergic reactions include bed bugs, fleas, mites, ticks, flies, midges, mosquitoes and spiders (including those not poisonous to humans). The insects are not shown to scale.

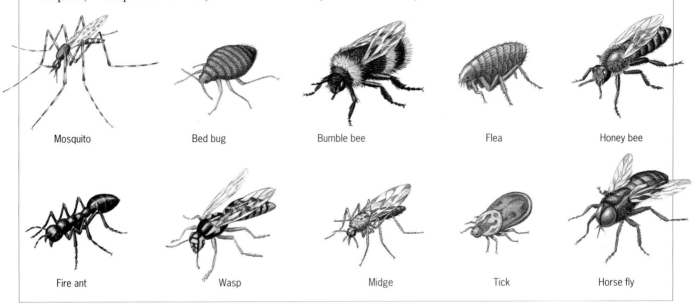

| Mosquito | Bed bug | Bumble bee | Flea | Honey bee |

| Fire ant | Wasp | Midge | Tick | Horse fly |

diarrhoea, accompanied by a feeling of impending doom. Severe anaphylaxis can cause breathing difficulties and collapse, and is an acute medical emergency. However, anaphylaxis responds well to the prompt administration of adrenaline, and patients at risk should carry adrenaline with them (see page 128).

Mild anaphylaxis tends to get worse on subsequent occasions, so people who have urticaria or angio-oedema that is becoming more severe on each occasion, are also often advised to carry adrenaline.

How do you know if you are at risk?

A previous reaction to an insect sting is the biggest risk factor for a serious allergic reaction. If you have never had a serious reaction before you probably do not need to worry, but if you have previously suffered a systemic reaction of any grade you should be extremely cautious.

But anaphylaxis is unpredictable and some of the people who die may have had no previous history of sting allergy. There is a blood test that can check for sensitivity to Hymenoptera venom, but a negative result does not totally exclude the possibility of a reaction and some people who test positive have previously shown no reaction to stings. If you are positive on testing, consider a course of venom immunotherapy which will reduce the potential severity of reactions.

Being stung frequently can increase the likelihood of hypersensitivity. On the other hand, if there are long intervals between stings a reaction may become less likely. This is because the level of IgE (the immunoglobin that causes an allergic response to insect stings – see Chapter 1) specific to that insect's venom will often fall over time.

WHAT IF YOU ARE STUNG?

Bee stings in particular are more dangerous as they impart a greater dose of venom than wasp and hornet stings (see page 124). Currently, the best advice to anyone who has previously suffered a systemic reaction to stings is to carry adrenaline with them at all times (see page 128). If stung, administer the adrenaline immediately and call for emergency medical help.

OTHER INSECTS THAT CAUSE ALLERGIC REACTIONS

Mosquito bites can cause swelling and irritation at the site of the bite, which can last for several days. This is more common in

First Aid for

Insect Allergies

Severe allergic reactions require immediate medical attention at hospital and an injection of adrenaline, but there are a variety of simple treatments you can use at home to help with minor reactions and irritation.

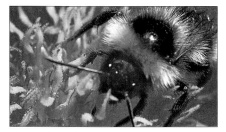

HONEY BEE
The honey bee, Apis mellifera, *can be found throughout Britain. It is one of many species of bee with a barbed sting.*

All stings cause pain, itching and swelling at the site of the sting – systemic reactions generally start within half an hour of the sting. If the stinger is left in the skin it must be removed using tweezers, the point of a needle or the back of a finger nail. Care is needed to avoid compressing the venom sac and injecting more venom into the skin.

TREATING LOCAL IRRITATION

If an insect bite or sting produces local irritation, swelling and pain, but not a more serious reaction, you can take paracetamol to relieve the pain and an antihistamine by mouth to relieve the irritation. Antihistamine creams may help.

Alternatively you could try a homeopathic remedy. If in doubt, always ask a qualified homeopathic physician for advice.

For bee or wasp stings they often prescribe one tablet of *Apis mel* every 15 minutes for an hour or so, depending on the severity of the sting.

For any puncture wounds or stings, take one tablet of *Ledum* (or one lid full of granules for infants) every 10–15 minutes for 3–4 doses, then one tablet every three hours until the pain subsides.

Homeopathic remedies are appropriate for minor reactions, but if there is any danger of a more serious reaction, get medical help.

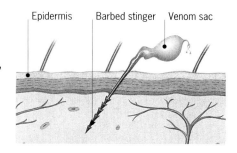

Epidermis   Barbed stinger   Venom sac

HOW A STING WORKS
Barbed stings are left in the skin of victims together with the venom sac, which continues to pump poison.

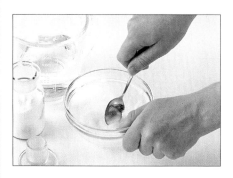

BEE STINGS
For bee stings an alternative treatment to antihistamines is a paste of water and sodium bicarbonate (baking soda) which should be applied to the site of the sting. A mouthwash of sodium bicarbonate (one teaspoon in a glass of water) makes a quick, soothing remedy for bee stings to the mouth, but these need proper medical attention immediately.

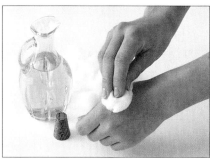

WASP STINGS
For wasp stings you can use plain cider vinegar. Do not confuse this treatment with baking soda for a bee sting. After applying treatment for either a wasp or bee sting, wrap a bag of ice in a towel and hold it over the site of the sting. Alternatively, a slice of raw onion held or bound over the site of the sting is an old folk remedy for wasp and bee stings.

ADRENALINE

If you know that you have a systemic allergy to stings, you should carry adrenaline with you at all times. If a serious reaction starts to happen, you must be given adrenaline (as an injection in the outer side of the thigh, or a spray to the inside of the mouth) and antihistamines immediately, then taken to an emergency medical centre (you may need more adrenaline). If adrenaline is not available it is essential that you seek medical help as a matter of extreme urgency.

children, but the reactions are hardly ever serious. However, in some parts of the world mosquitoes carry malarial parasites which can cause allergic reactions (in addition to malaria). Certain antihistamines, such as Cetirizine, can suppress the allergic symptoms if taken immediately after a bite or in anticipation of being bitten.

Other biting insects which usually cause only moderate reactions in allergic individuals, but can cause anaphylaxis in rare cases, include horse, deer and black flies, midges, fleas, ticks, lice and some spiders. Bed bugs (Cimex species) can cause large, raised weals in rare cases. There is no specific treatment apart from antihistamine, which will reduce the itching. Try not to scratch insect bites.

A particular problem with ticks is that they bury their mouth parts in the skin when they bite. If a biting tick is not removed with extreme care, the mouthparts can be left behind and cause irritation and even infections. Try applying a layer of nail varnish to the exposed body of the tick, which causes it to loosen its grip, making it easier to remove safely. Alternatively, ticks can be burnt off with the lit end of a cigarette.

AVOIDING BITES AND STINGS

There are certain scents and clothing which attract stinging insects and others which protect against them. There are also certain places where insects are most likely to be found, and certain situations where they are more likely to become aggressive. The chart below describes some of the most common risk factors and what to do about them.

If you are attacked

If you spot a swarm keep well away and notify a local bee-keeper or your local borough pest control officer. Do not panic: swarms of bees are usually less aggressive than single bees because they've eaten all the honey they can carry, which makes them relatively docile. Try to move slowly without any sudden movements until you are a safe distance away. If you are attacked, cover your head with your arms or a piece of clothing; bees and wasps instinctively go for the dark patches on faces – the mouth, eyes, nostrils and ears. If you come across a nest, on no account disturb it. Move slowly away, and phone the fire brigade, local bee-keeper or the local borough pest control officer to come and remove it.

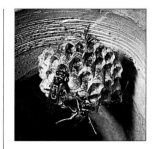

WASPS' NEST
Common spots for wasps' nests are under the eaves of houses and in trees, including old tree trunks. Generally, wasps in temperate countries only form nests during the spring, summer and autumn. During the winter, the queen hibernates and the other wasps die off.

PREVENTING INSECT BITES AND STINGS

As with any allergy, prevention is the best cure, so avoiding insect bites and stings in the first place is the best way to spare yourself a nasty reaction. The chart below describes some of the factors and situations that can attract or aggravate insects, especially wasps, hornets and bees, together with tips and strategies to help you minimise the risk of being stung or bitten.

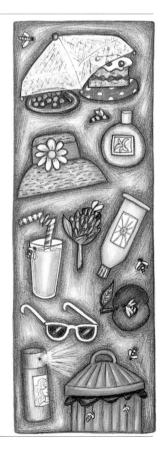

RISK FACTOR	DO'S AND DON'TS
Scents	Perfumes, hairsprays, strongly scented sun creams and shampoos – all attract wasps and other Vespids. They are also attracted to sweat and the carbon dioxide in a person's breath, so take care when exercising outside.
Movements	Avoid sudden movements when approached by a stinging insect.
Being inside	Keep windows shut or covered with fine netting, and food and bins covered up.
Being outside	Avoid orchards with fallen ripe fruit as these attract wasps. Do not disturb fallen tree trunks as wasps and bees are likely to nest in these. Bees are attracted to clover in the grass and also nest in the ground. Keep food covered if eating outside, and avoid places where animals are fed.
Clothing	Avoid loose fitting or brightly coloured clothes: neutral coloured, green or brown clothes are best. Stay covered up while gardening, with long trousers and long-sleeved shirts. A hat and gloves provide extra protection. Wear gloves and helmet when riding a motorbike. If riding a bicycle try to keep your mouth shut and wear sunglasses. Never walk barefoot outside.

UNUSUAL ALLERGIES

Some very unusual skin allergies have been recorded – allergies to substances that are important or even vital to everyday life and as varied as water, seminal fluid and even other people.

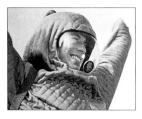

STAYING INSIDE
Some unlucky allergy sufferers develop so many sensitivities that they are only well in special allergen-free environments, as in the 1977 TV film, The Boy In The Plastic Bubble, *starring John Travolta, pictured here in an environmental isolation suit. The allergies and sensitivities themselves may not be unusual, but having so many of them is, fortunately, rare.*

In theory, you can become allergic to practically anything, and there are many unusual allergies that can be debilitating and even life-threatening for the sufferers.

For instance, you may have symptoms when you are with certain people. The most likely cause will be their perfume, washing powder or pets. Allergies to people themselves are rare, and are caused either by skin particles, hair or fluid. Reactions to hair and skin particles are more likely in people already suffering from eczema.

Some women may be allergic to seminal fluid, resulting in hives or even, very rarely, anaphylaxis. Reactions can be avoided if the male withdraws before ejaculation or by using a condom. Some men react to feminine hygiene sprays used by their partner prior to intercourse.

Both partners can develop skin reactions to propylene glycol, an ingredient of some lubricating agents. Reactions to rubber diaphragms and rubber latex condom sheaths may occur in the vulva, vagina and penis. Polyurethane condoms are available for those allergic to rubber, but some people are allergic to these as well.

Vulval inflammation may also be caused by douches, feminine hygiene sprays or skin medications. Allergic reactions may result from vaginal spermicides, hair removing agents, soaps, bubble baths, some sanitary towels and the residues of chemicals left on the hands.

TEMPERATURE SENSITIVITY

In rare circumstances sunlight can cause a rapid onset of hives. The electromagnetic radiation in the sun's rays causes the mast cells in the skin to discharge their inflammatory contents (including histamine).

Cold produced by low air temperatures or contact with ice or snow can also cause hives. If your whole body is exposed, for instance if you fall into icy water, a state similar to anaphylactic shock can occur, which is thought to be due to excess histamine production. Seek immediate medical attention.

WATER SENSITIVITY

Chemicals in tap water may cause allergic reactions. Chlorine in swimming pools can be a problem; lesser concentrations are present in tap water. Filtered or bottled water for drinking and washing may be necessary.

There is a vary rare condition called aquagenic urticaria in which the skin develops hives when exposed to any water: tap water, distilled water, and even the person's own sweat or tears. This reaction is caused by the chemical acetylcholine which is released when water touches the skin. The drug scopolamine is used to treat the condition.

FILTERING WATER

People sensitive to water contaminants may be better using filtered water for drinking or washing. A jug filter may be adequate but a quality plumbed-in filter is usually more effective.

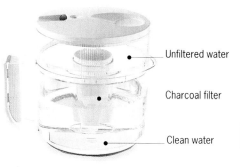

Unfiltered water

Charcoal filter

Clean water

ALLERGY-FREE WATER
A jug filter should remove contaminants such as chlorine, nitrates, pesticides and lead, and may even help soften hard water.

ANAPHYLAXIS

Sudden onset of severe allergic symptoms – a feeling of doom, itchiness, swelling, racing pulse and difficult breathing – signals a serious anaphylactic attack. This is a medical emergency.

Those most at risk of very severe anaphylaxis (anaphylactic shock) are people who have previously had a severe reaction to an allergen, but anyone could suffer an attack, and not everyone has worsening mild symptoms to warn them. How can you recognise the danger signs if you've never had a reaction before?

SYMPTOMS

The first symptom is often a foreboding that all is not well. This is followed – particularly if a food is the cause – by immediate burning, irritation or itching of the lips, mouth and throat. These lead in turn to swelling (oedema) of the mouth, face, tongue and throat, swelling of the airways causing breathing problems, skin reactions and stomach problems like cramps or nausea. Blood pressure drops, and weakness and unconsciousness may result.

In children, the first sign is often a change in the colour of the skin, blotchiness of the chest or purple fingers which, after going pale (blanching) when squeezed, do not recover their colour quickly.

Death can be caused either by suffocation because the throat is blocked by swelling, or from heart failure because of the fall in blood pressure. It should be stressed that these are very rare manifestations of an untreated severe reaction. Less severe cases may recover spontaneously, while prompt treatment ensures recovery for others.

COMMON TRIGGERS

Penicillin is now the most common cause of anaphylaxis, followed by foods such as peanuts, fish and shellfish, then wasp and bee stings. Other causes include vaccines, immunotherapy, blood transfusions, natural rubber latex, and in some cases, exercise. Although anaphylaxis is unpredictable, it is more likely to occur in patients who have

had severe urticaria. Other risk factors include older age, asthma (especially in children) and taking beta-blockers (prescribed for heart problems and other conditions). Also, people who are atopic – that is, people who have a generally high level of IgE and are thus highly sensitive to allergenic substances – may be at slightly greater risk than most individuals.

Exercise-induced anaphylaxis

In rare cases anaphylaxis may be provoked by exercise. Sometimes this only happens with a combination of exercise and having eaten a specific food a few hours beforehand. In such cases, neither of these factors brings on an attack on its own. Other factors which may contribute to the onset of exercise-induced anaphylaxis are exercising in an extremely hot or cold environment or in high humidity, exercising while

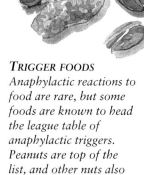

TRIGGER FOODS
Anaphylactic reactions to food are rare, but some foods are known to head the league table of anaphylactic triggers. Peanuts are top of the list, and other nuts also rank highly.

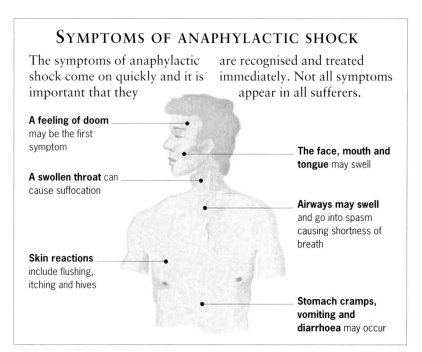

SYMPTOMS OF ANAPHYLACTIC SHOCK

The symptoms of anaphylactic shock come on quickly and it is important that they are recognised and treated immediately. Not all symptoms appear in all sufferers.

A feeling of doom may be the first symptom

A swollen throat can cause suffocation

Skin reactions include flushing, itching and hives

The face, mouth and tongue may swell

Airways may swell and go into spasm causing shortness of breath

Stomach cramps, vomiting and diarrhoea may occur

TREATING ANAPHYLAXIS

The most important aspect of treating anaphylaxis is to act quickly, give adrenaline and antihistamines and call medical help. The sufferer should be laid flat and then have the feet raised, unless they are having breathing difficulties.

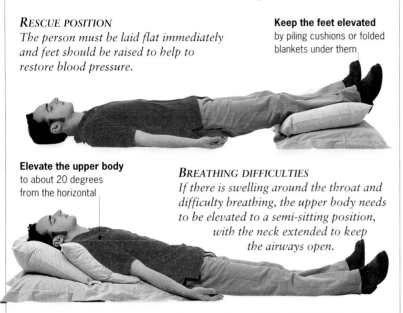

RESCUE POSITION
The person must be laid flat immediately and feet should be raised to help to restore blood pressure.

Keep the feet elevated
by piling cushions or folded blankets under them

Elevate the upper body
to about 20 degrees from the horizontal

BREATHING DIFFICULTIES
If there is swelling around the throat and difficulty breathing, the upper body needs to be elevated to a semi-sitting position, with the neck extended to keep the airways open.

menstruating, drug ingestion before exercise (taking aspirin, for instance) and hot showers after exercise.

Vaccine anaphylaxis

Anaphylactic reactions to vaccines are also very rare and unpredictable, and may occur in people who have no known risk factors. During the 1994 measles and rubella immunisation campaign in the UK, 81 cases of anaphylaxis were reported out of about 8 million children immunised, and there were no deaths. Doctors keep adrenaline to hand when undertaking immunisations.

Latex anaphylaxis

A very small but increasing number of people are extremely allergic to natural rubber latex. Those particularly at risk are people who work in the rubber industry and medical personnel who use rubber gloves – the allergens may be present in the powder in which the gloves are coated. Other sources of contact with latex include: comforters (dummies), rubber toys or balloons, rubber gloves for housework or rubber condoms.

Anyone who has suffered acute latex allergy before must warn their doctor, gynaecologist or dentist before undergoing any examination or operation, in case the practitioner uses rubber latex gloves. Non-latex alternatives are available.

TREATMENT

Fast treatment is essential. At the onset of an anaphylactic reaction, the sufferer should be laid flat and, most importantly, given adrenaline. Anyone who knows that they are susceptible to anaphylactic shock should always carry their own adrenaline in a pre-loaded syringe for self-injection or as a spray. The best forms are called EPIPEN and ANAPEN – these are easy to use, and come in child and adult sizes. The adrenaline should be injected in the side of the leg.

Some patients are prescribed an adrenaline inhaler instead. In an emergency these are used to spray onto the inside of the cheek, using at least 20 sprays for an adult. This is less intimidating than self-injection. Sufferers should also carry antihistamine for emergencies, provided they can swallow.

An emergency adrenaline shot is only the first step in the treatment of anaphylaxis. Further treatment with more adrenaline and other drugs is often essential. Anyone who has suffered an anaphylactic attack should seek urgent medical attention, even if they appear to be recovering. Occasionally patients suffer a relapse as late as the next day, and so require further treatment.

PRECAUTIONS

People who know they are susceptible to anaphylaxis should carry a warning card or wear a pendant with the details of their allergy. They should carry a prescribed emergency kit at all times and should get a trainer kit so that both the patient and the relatives can learn how to use it. A child's teacher should be vigilant – children may be offered allergenic foods by their friends without realising the danger. Everyone should know where to find the adrenaline and how to give it in an emergency.

> **WARNING**
> *Adrenaline may be dangerous for people with heart disease. For children, a teacher or school nurse must be trained to recognise the symptoms of anaphylaxis and how to give adrenaline.*

CHAPTER 8

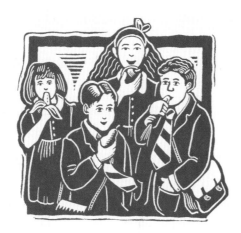

CHILDREN AND ALLERGY

From simple coughs and sleepless nights to behavioural disorders and educational underachievement, the symptoms of allergy can make a child's life – and that of the parents – unbearable. If doctors and parents know what to look for and how to deal with it, they can make a huge difference to a child's health, mental well-being and future.

PREVENTION OF ALLERGIES

Taking special care in the two years from the time that you decide to have a baby until your baby is one year old can help to avoid years of caring for a child with allergies.

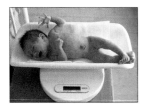

BIRTH WEIGHT AND ALLERGY
Good nutrition for the mother increases the chance that her baby will grow to a good size and that the pregnancy will continue to full term. There is evidence of an association between low birth weight and the development of asthma and possibly other allergies.

It is known that a tendency to develop allergies runs in families. Research indicates that this tendency has a complex pattern of inheritance and there is little likelihood of screening tests for susceptibility to allergies being developed in the short term.

To reduce the chance of having a baby prone to allergies it is advisable to start planning at least three months before you become pregnant. There is growing evidence that the parents' nutrition, lifestyle and environment during this time can influence the later development of allergies in their child.

DIETARY FACTORS

It is essential that the mother pays close attention to her nutrition from three months before conception until at least the end of breastfeeding. Prospective mothers should not be underweight, or miss meals. Dietary trace elements, particularly zinc, selenium and magnesium, and certain vitamins, mainly the B group, have a major effect on the development and functioning of the immune system. Significant amounts of these essential nutrients are found in fresh meats, fish and green vegetables, but many people are deficient in some of these nutrients so it might be wise to get advice from a nutritionist or to take a supplement specially designed by experts for use in pregnancy, such as one produced for Foresight, the Society for the Promotion of Preconceptual Care. It is important to take good advice – high-dose supplements can be harmful.

This dietary advice does not just apply to mothers – a man's sperm quality may be adversely affected by poor nutrition. Men

NUTRITION IN PREGNANCY

Throughout pregnancy and when breastfeeding a mother should eat a very varied diet, avoiding large amounts of any one food, especially dairy products. Evidence shows that foreign proteins, such as casein in cow's milk, can cross the placenta from the mother's bloodstream to the foetus' and can get into breast milk.

BABY FOOD
Eat a variety of healthy foods, avoiding the main food allergy triggers.

Placenta Placental barrier Maternal blood Foetal blood

The placental barrier
In the placenta, nutrients and oxygen pass from the mother's blood into the foetus'. The two bloodstreams are separated by a membrane which keeps germs from infecting the foetal blood, but may allow some allergens to pass.

need to start preparing early as sperm is most at risk three months before it matures. A few months of nutritional 'therapy' may be needed to put right any problems.

Mother-child transfer of allergens

The developing immune system in foetuses and babies under three months old is still learning to distinguish between its own tissue, which it needs to tolerate, and foreign material which it needs to reject. During this time it is particularly vulnerable to high levels of exposure to foreign proteins, which can disturb and interfere with this learning process. This in turn can cause the infant's immune system to become hypersensitive – the condition known as atopy.

For reasons that are not entirely clear, this response can happen with any foreign protein but is particularly likely to happen with pollen or dust, and with milk if it forms a large part of the mother's diet.

Breastfeeding

A baby's intestines have a role in determining whether or not the child develops allergies. For at least three months after birth a baby's gut continues to develop. Breast milk is designed to help mature the gut and reduce the absorption of proteins which might lead to allergies. Ideally it should be the sole source of nutrition, with any weaning delayed until at least four months. Solids should be introduced between four and six months, according to the baby's appetite, but avoiding the most common allergy triggers. Breast milk is the best milk to use until at least one year old.

Many mothers give up breastfeeding needlessly. This is sometimes because of the growth and behaviour pattern of breastfed babies. They often take more, but shorter, feeds than bottle-fed babies and they may not gain weight as rapidly in the first few months. These features can cause anxiety that the baby is not being satisfied by the breast milk. Get the advice of your midwife, health visitor or local breastfeeding support group before reacting to what is a normal pattern of feeding for a breastfed baby.

LIFESTYLE FACTORS

Stress is known to affect the body's immune responses, including allergic reactions (see page 41). It also increases the risk of problems in pregnancy that may lead to low birth weight: both foetuses and babies are able to perceive stress in their environment, and may react adversely.

Relaxation

Ideally a mother should be as relaxed as possible throughout pregnancy and during a baby's first year of life. This is a difficult demand to meet, as pregnancy, childbirth and caring for an infant can all cause considerable stress. Reducing stress levels involves planning ahead carefully, and perhaps using some relaxation techniques, such as yoga, aromatherapy or t'ai chi.

Smoking

Tobacco smoke greatly increases the risk of asthma in infancy, as well as increasing the likelihood of premature birth and low birth weight. Evidence from a 1978 American study of more than two thousand patients, and from a 1988 Swedish study published in the *Archives of Diseases in Childhood*, shows that tobacco smoke helps to 'switch on' the allergy system.

ENVIRONMENTAL FACTORS

Heavy exposure to certain products in the atmosphere plays a major role in setting the immune system on the path to allergy. Evidence particularly implicates high levels of infant exposure to house dust mites, moulds and cat dander (flakes of skin).

Protective measures for children are essentially the same as those for adults (see Chapter 3). Well ventilated houses, kept at an even temperature of 18–21°C (65–70°F), with electric cookers, bare floors, washable rugs and curtains, and a minimum of synthetic fabrics, provide the ideal low-allergen environment, keeping dust mites, moulds and chemicals to a minimum. A handy tip for keeping children's cuddly toys, pillows and duvets free of dust mites, without using toxic anti-mite chemicals, is to put them in the deep freeze for 12 hours every fortnight.

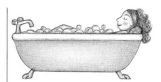

RELAXING AROMAS
Aromatherapy oils added to bath water can be an aid to relaxation, but some oils should be avoided by pregnant women – in particular sage, basil, myrrh, thyme and marjoram. Lavender oil is safe and relaxing.

THE BIG CHILL
Keep down the dust mite population of your child's soft toys with a spell in the freezer.

MANAGING YOUR CHILD'S ALLERGY

Successfully identifying and managing a child's allergy involves striking a delicate balance between changing and restricting the child's environment and minimising his or her distress.

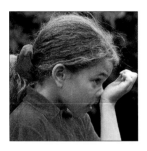

ALLERGIC SALUTE
Allergic rhinitis can cause a persistently itchy, blocked or runny nose. Children whose noses are constantly dripping develop a habitual response, known as an 'allergic salute'. They push up the end of their noses to wipe away mucus and relieve itches.

How can you tell if your child's illness or discomfort is due to an allergic reaction? How can you find out what he or she is allergic to? Parents should be aware of some key signs.

IDENTIFYING YOUR CHILD'S ALLERGY
If your child is continually ill with varying disorders, and especially if allergies run in your family, you should suspect allergies. Before taking action, however, it is essential to check with your doctor to make sure that there is no other condition present that needs a different form of treatment.

WHICH CHILDREN ARE MORE LIKELY TO BE AFFECTED?
Because susceptibility to allergies has a strong genetic element, children with a family history of allergies are a definite risk group. In childhood, boys are more likely to develop allergies than girls. This is particularly the case for attention deficit disorder which is an increasingly common symptom of hidden food allergy in children.

KEY MARKERS FOR ALLERGY
Allergies may cause multiple symptoms, affecting different systems of the body. The presence of multiple symptoms is one of the

SYMPTOMS OF ALLERGY AND INTOLERANCE

There is an extensive range of symptoms that can be related to allergies and intolerances to foods or agents in the environment. It should be stressed that many of these symptoms may have causes other than allergy or intolerance.

SYMPTOM GROUP	ACTUAL CONDITIONS
Gut problems	Diarrhoea, constipation, recurrent stomach pains, colic in babies, feeding difficulties, itching anus, recurrent vomiting or feeling of sickness, mouth ulcers, poor appetite, food cravings
Brain/mood problems	Recurrent headaches or migraines, dizziness, poor concentration, hyperactivity, fidgeting, night waking, unexplained temper tantrums, attention deficit disorder, depression, fits, restlessness, disturbed sleep, balance problems, persistent lethargy
Urinary/genital systems	Vaginal itching/discharge, sore genitals, frequent urinating, bed-wetting
Breathing problems	Blocked or runny nose, nose bleeds, pain in the front of the face (sinus pain), snoring, catarrh, glue ear, wheezing and asthma
Skin problems	Eczema, recurrent allergy rashes, itchiness of the skin, increased sweating
Joints and muscles	Recurrent joint pains and juvenile arthritis, muscle aching, muscle weakness, cramps
General	Increased thirst, recurrent unexplained high temperatures, swollen lymph glands, nightmares, talking/walking in sleep, obesity, weight loss

key markers that an allergy underlies a child's condition. If a child is affected by only one or two of these symptoms it is unlikely that the problems are related to allergy, although some conditions such as asthma or migraine may occur in isolation.

Food allergies and intolerances have their own particular markers – excessive thirst is the best indicator, being present in 95 per cent of cases, and craving for a particular food is often a useful clue. Conversely, an aversion to the taste or smell of a food may indicate a food to avoid.

Diagnosis

The initial diagnosis of allergy as a cause of a child's symptoms is based on recognising the symptom patterns described above. After this the same procedures – often laborious and inconvenient – must be applied as with adults (see Chapter 1). Laboratory tests, such as a RAST test, may be useful for confirming some inhalant allergies, but are of limited help. For full and proper diagnosis, a detailed history is essential. This may need to be followed by precautions against house dust mites, moulds or animals, or elimination diets and food challenges. These are the only truly reliable methods.

TREATING A CHILD'S ALLERGY

Avoiding allergens may require major changes in lifestyle and diet. It can be enormously worth while but for a child the restrictions can be distressing, socially damaging and very difficult to put into practice. This can be counterproductive because stressed and upset children are far more prone to allergic attacks – parents should try to avoid doing more harm than good.

YOUR CHILD'S ENVIRONMENT

Most of the principles of environmental management for adults also apply to allergic children. It is essential to consider all the environments in which a child will spend time, including home, school, with grandparents or at a separated parent's house.

Planning major changes

When contemplating major changes in your environment it is essential to plan ahead. For instance, if moving house check the area thoroughly from the point of view of an allergy sufferer and try to stay nearby for a trial period. If planning to get a pet, try to arrange for your child to visit the shop or owner daily for three weeks before buying, so you can check for an allergic reaction.

Airborne allergens

House dust mites, moulds and dander from pets are the major airborne allergens, with pollen becoming more important as a child grows older. Chemical allergens, such as formaldehyde, are particularly implicated in asthma and allergic rhinitis. Even if your child's allergy is to a food rather than an airborne allergen, it is still important to reduce his or her exposure to airborne allergens because they increase the total 'allergen load'. This means that they increase the stress on an allergic child's already overstretched immune system.

YOUR CHILD'S DIET

If it is established that your child has a food allergy or intolerance, then his or her diet will need to be modified. What degree of change do you need to implement?

Is total avoidance necessary?

Some children with allergies are unable to tolerate even minute amounts of a trigger food and will have to avoid it completely – for instance, a child who develops anaphylaxis after exposure to a trace of peanut.

There are many other children, however, who have a degree of tolerance to a food, allowing them to eat small amounts occasionally without developing severe symptoms. Often children start off very sensitive and develop tolerance over time.

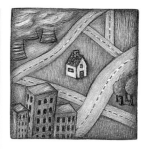

NASTY NEIGHBOURS
If you are serious about avoiding sources of trouble, check out a new area thoroughly before moving there. Avoid obvious problem spots such as chemical plants or fields that are sprayed.

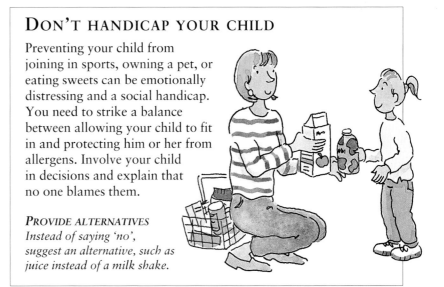

DON'T HANDICAP YOUR CHILD

Preventing your child from joining in sports, owning a pet, or eating sweets can be emotionally distressing and a social handicap. You need to strike a balance between allowing your child to fit in and protecting him or her from allergens. Involve your child in decisions and explain that no one blames them.

PROVIDE ALTERNATIVES
Instead of saying 'no', suggest an alternative, such as juice instead of a milk shake.

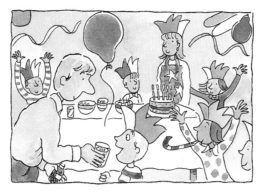

Getting your child's help

Successfully modifying your child's diet depends on getting his or her cooperation. This means that you must explain why the changes are being made. You may even have to allow a lapse in the diet, so that your child starts to recognise the association between what he or she eats and the unpleasant consequences.

For some children who can't avoid 'cheating' occasionally, a preventative oral preparation of disodium cromoglycate, taken just prior to the lapse, may reduce the reaction.

Balancing your child's diet

Simply excluding additives (see Chapter 4) from a child's diet can be done without any harm to nutrition, but more complex diets may require the advice of a dietitian or nutritionist to help you to ensure that the diet has no deficiencies in vitamins, minerals or other nutrients.

ANTIFUNGAL THERAPY

This is a controversial approach to the management of allergies, but some specialists argue that antifungal therapy is a helpful alternative to trying to keep a child on a permanently restricted diet.

What is it?

Antifungal therapy is based on the theory that yeast and fungal microorganisms in the gut cause the symptoms of hidden food allergy and intolerance, either by acting as allergens themselves, or by producing toxic fermentation products. The therapy is based on a diet involving the exclusion of sugars, yeast extracts and fermented products.

In addition to these dietary controls, a naturopath might use herbal medicines, such as garlic, supplements of vitamins B and C and live yoghurt or cultures of friendly bacteria (see page 89).

Who can it help?

This therapy is most likely to be effective in children who have a history of frequent episodes of thrush (Candida albicans infection), who have had repeated antibiotic treatment, or whose parents are prone to thrush. It is important for the doctor or therapist to confirm that yeast, and not bacterial, overgrowth is responsible for the problems. This can be done with some simple laboratory investigations.

The role of antifungal drugs

Although a very strict diet is often recommended for adults, many children respond to a less strenuous dietary regime combined with treatment with an anti-fungal drug. If the treatment is effective it may need to be continued for several months.

A naturopath would favour a gentler, natural antifungal preparation of caprylic acid, based on coconut oil.

WHAT THE CHILD CAN DO

Many children will be the best guardians of their own diet once they are aware of what makes them feel unwell. Older children may be able to keep their own records of symptoms to help with the identification of triggers. Children are also often good at avoiding environments that don't suit them – many children are the strongest critics of their parents' smoking habits.

The most difficult group of children are those whose need for a special diet is not identified until they are ten years old. By this age they are very resistant to change. Early identification of children with allergies and intolerances is thus very important.

Pathway to health

Excluding cow's milk is a common anti-allergy dietary measure, but it often causes parents anxiety over whether their child will suffer from a deficiency of calcium. Soya milk fortified with calcium, or calcium supplements from your doctor or a pharmacy can be used. For children over 18 months old, goat's or sheep's milk are an acceptable substitute, if tolerated. Always check with a doctor or dietitian before making major changes in your child's diet.

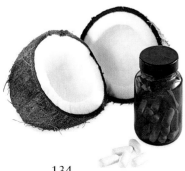

Easing a Child's Asthma Attack with

Relaxation

The most effective way to help a child in the event of an asthma attack is to be prepared for one before it happens. Knowing what to do and when will reassure and calm both you and your child, which could be your most important contribution.

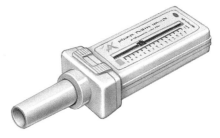

PEAK FLOW METER
A peak flow meter is an easy-to-use tool for measuring the degree of constriction of the bronchi. Changes can serve as early warning of an attack.

During an asthma attack the airways become constricted (bronchospasm) and fill with mucus, so a child will have difficulty breathing out, rather than in. Nonetheless, the worst thing the child can do is panic, which may worsen the attack. Stay calm and reassure the child – the presence of a relaxed, confident adult may be the most effective calming influence a child can have. Assess the severity of the attack – a severe attack will require medical attention, so before progressing further with self-help efforts check for some warning signs. The most obvious is cyanosis – a blue tinge to the lips and tongue. A peak flow meter can help in gauging severity. If you suspect that the attack is severe, get medical help as soon as possible, either from a doctor or at the nearest Accident and Emergency department. While waiting for help, get the child into the correct position, and keep him or her calm. Clear the room and minimise distractions. Prevent fumes or smoke from worsening the child's condition. Get the child to breathe slowly, concentrating on breathing out. After an acute attack, even one that was successfully controlled, you should have your child checked by a doctor or local hospital to see if additional treatment is required.

POSITION YOUR CHILD CORRECTLY

During an asthma attack, get your child to sit up and lean forward slightly, ideally with something to lean on. Don't make him or her lie down.

LEAN FORWARD
In an asthma attack a child uses the muscles around the chest to help with breathing. Leaning forward slightly helps these to work.

Soothe the child with words of encouragement and try to remain as calm as possible.

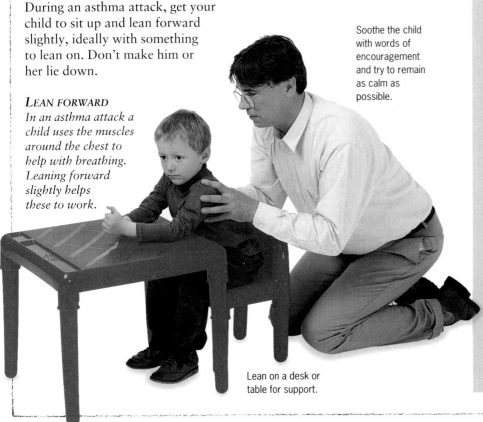

Lean on a desk or table for support.

MEDICATION

Administering medication promptly and accurately is crucial in controlling an asthma attack. Familiarise yourself with your child's different medications, and make sure everyone in the household knows where they are kept. The most common medications are salbutamol (Ventolin) and terbutaline (Bricanyl) – given as dry powder, or by aerosol or nebuliser. It is very difficult to take an overdose of this medication, and in an attack a child may require several times the usual treatment dose, so err on the side of giving more rather than less. While waiting for medical assistance a child may need reliever medication repeated every 15 minutes.

HYPERACTIVITY AND FOOD ALLERGIES

A disorder often linked with childhood allergy is hyperactivity, or attention deficit disorder. It can cause emotional damage and hinder a child's education, but may be helped by changes in diet.

SYMPTOMS OF ADHD

Children suffering from ADHD commonly exhibit symptoms such as:

▶ *Hyperactivity and excitability, talking too fast.*

▶ *Constant fidgeting.*

▶ *Inability to concentrate, frequent shifts of attention, easily distracted.*

▶ *Doing badly at school, disruptive and difficult.*

▶ *Unpredictable, explosive mood changes.*

▶ *Being aggressive, quick to anger and easily depressed.*

▶ *Being clumsy and poorly coordinated.*

▶ *Poor self-image.*

▶ *Disturbed sleep.*

▶ *Constant thirst.*

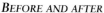

BEFORE AND AFTER
One sign of improvement in hyperactive children is better drawing skills, reflecting improved concentration and dexterity.

Hyperactivity is just one aspect of a syndrome known variously as attention deficit hyperactivity disorder (ADHD), attention deficit spectrum, hyperkinetic syndrome or minimal brain dysfunction. All describe essentially the same syndrome with a range of related symptoms and only minor differences.

HOW IS THE SYNDROME DIAGNOSED?

Media interest in ADHD has given the impression that it is a well-defined disorder for which there is a single diagnosis. This is not the case. Many people prefer to use the term 'Attention Deficit Spectrum' to reflect that the disorder can vary in severity and range of symptoms. In practice the grouping of symptoms associated with ADHD can be attributed to at least 14 possible diagnoses, each needing a different approach. High amongst these possibilities are food intolerance, food allergy (in particular to additives) or a nutritional deficiency. Although powerful drugs are available for controlling the disorder (and are widely used in the United States), it makes sense to exclude

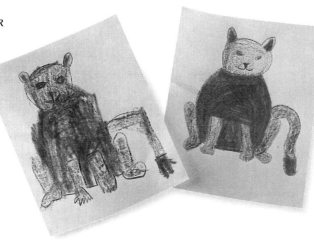

these possibilities before risking side effects from a drug therapy which does not address the root cause of the problem.

Children who are likely to benefit from dietary treatment can usually be identified using the same criteria as those for any food allergy or intolerance – by observing the symptoms, the timing and combination of symptoms, and the response of the affected child to an elimination diet.

WHAT PROOF IS THERE THAT ALLERGIES ARE INVOLVED?

The role played by food allergy in the behavioural problems of hyperactive children is one of the most controversial topics in medicine. There are still many sceptics, despite some excellent studies from the Great Ormond Street Children's Hospital, in London, which have established the benefits that dietary treatment can produce in some hyperactive children.

These studies found that severely hyperactive children showed marked improvement after the introduction of a 'few foods' diet (a diet more strict than the Stone Age diet, excluding most common allergenic foods).

Some of the children were given double-blind food challenges to see whether any particular food trigger could be identified. A statistically significant proportion were shown to have increased symptoms after such challenges, proving the involvement of food.

There is continuing debate over how many hyperactive children can be helped through diet, although a 1994 American study in the *Annals of Allergy* suggested that 74 per cent of children referred to a clinic with ADHD could be helped by dietary change.

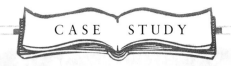

CASE STUDY

The Hyperactive Child

Hyperactivity is just one aspect of a debilitating condition called the attention deficit spectrum, or the attention deficit hyperactivity disorder (ADHD). Children suffering from this disorder generally have high levels of nervous activity – they have difficulty at school, get into fights, and find it impossible to sit still at home.

Christopher is five years old and has a history of chronic medical complaints. He has had a constant runny nose and constipation for at least two years, and does not sleep well. His school complained of his frequent misbehaviour in class and his poor standard of speaking and drawing. His mother took him to see the family doctor because of these behavioural problems. The doctor noticed that Christopher looked unwell, with dark rings under his eyes, but that he was full of energy and constantly on the go – climbing onto chairs, picking things up and then dropping them – and easily distracted. The doctor also noted that Christopher continually sucked on a carton of blackcurrant juice and was perpetually thirsty.

WHAT CHRISTOPHER'S MOTHER SHOULD DO

The doctor had seen this combination of symptoms before, and recognised that Christopher had the condition ADHD. Because of the particular symptoms, the doctor suspected that the condition might be caused by food allergies and suggested that Christopher's mother try keeping him on a special elimination diet. This cut out the foods and drinks that Christopher craved most, together with foods high in additives and added sugar, and common allergenic culprits such as milk, wheat and eggs. If his symptoms improved, they would then try some food challenges to identify exactly which foods were responsible for the condition.

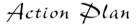

HEALTH
Food allergies can cause various chronic conditions, including bowel problems and runny nose. These can act as markers for allergic disorders.

DIET
Milk, wheat and eggs are common allergy triggers. Additives such as flavourings or colourings, together with high levels of refined sugar, are particularly implicated in ADHD.

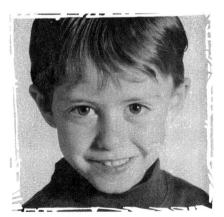

CHILDREN
Bad behaviour together with other symptoms may indicate a food allergy or intolerance.

Action Plan

DIET
Adopt a special diet: stop eating sweets and drinking soft drinks and juices. Cut out milk, wheat and eggs.

CHILDREN
Tell teachers, grandparents and the parents of the child's friends about the special diet, and make sure they know how important it is to stick to it.

HEALTH
Keep a diary of symptoms, situations and foods to identify triggers that should be avoided.

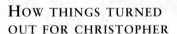

HOW THINGS TURNED OUT FOR CHRISTOPHER

After three weeks on the elimination diet, Christopher's nose stopped running and his constipation cleared up. Food challenges showed he was allergic to soft drinks and wheat. His sleep improved, as did his behaviour at home and at school, and he was able to concentrate and interact with other children. His teachers were very pleased with his new attentiveness, and reported that his speech and drawing skills were improving rapidly.

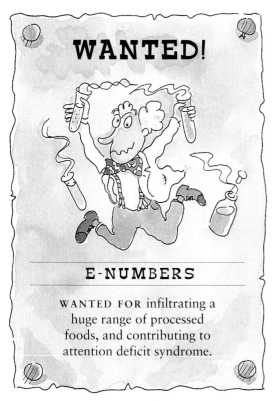

WANTED!

E-NUMBERS

WANTED FOR infiltrating a huge range of processed foods, and contributing to attention deficit syndrome.

PSYCHOLOGICAL FACTORS

In many cases where children demonstrate hyperactivity, impaired concentration, learning deficits and difficult behaviour there is also evidence of poor parenting and poor parent-child relationships. But these parenting problems may be a result rather than a cause of difficulties: many children with a hidden food allergy or intolerance will have been difficult from early infancy, presenting their parents with a child who cries a lot, perpetually disturbs their sleep, and who does not seem to give any positive feedback, such as reciprocating their affection. Inevitably this will affect the parents, impairing the process of attachment that is essential to good parent-child relationships. This is why it is important to recognise a child who is suffering from ADHD caused by food allergy or intolerance at the earliest possible stage, before any lasting damage occurs.

HYPERACTIVITY, STRESS AND CHILDREN

Being diagnosed as having ADHD, and then avoiding 'forbidden' foodstuffs, can take its toll on a child. In addition, prior to treatment, the ADHD may have caused difficulties within the family, and educational underachievement and low self-esteem in the child. Thus the problems created by ADHD may continue to cause emotional problems even after successful treatment – professionals call these secondary emotional difficulties. This produces more stress and emotional disturbance for the child, making him or her even more vulnerable to allergy.

Getting support

Parents and schools need to work together to help a child adapt to dietary restrictions, and this may be hindered if teachers or family and relatives are sceptical. A supportive report from a doctor or other specialist may help to convince people that they need to be positive about changes to a child's diet.

Managing stress

Avoiding situations which provoke anxiety is one way of reducing your child's stress, but this is not always possible. A more flexible approach is to help your child learn how to manage stressful situations. This may require counselling or the development of special coping skills and strategies.

ADHD AND FAMILY DYNAMICS

The symptoms of ADHD interact with psychological and emotional factors within the family. If left untreated, these problems can feed back on one another, causing a negative spiral of worsening behavioural and emotional difficulties.

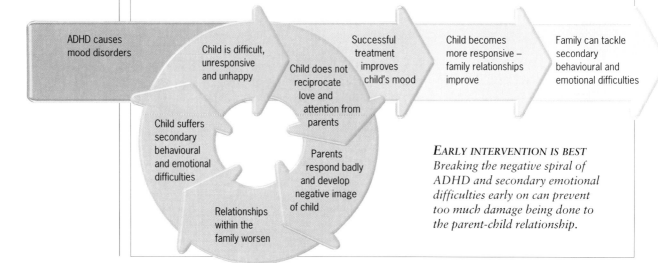

EARLY INTERVENTION IS BEST
Breaking the negative spiral of ADHD and secondary emotional difficulties early on can prevent too much damage being done to the parent-child relationship.

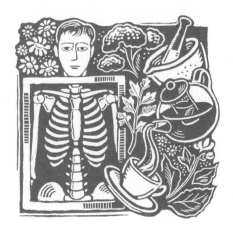

CHAPTER 9

A DIRECTORY OF ALLERGIC DISORDERS

Allergic reactions have been implicated as the hidden cause of a host of conditions, many of which are chronic and incapacitating. Avoidance measures and elimination diets can often help where doctors have excluded other causes and are at a loss as to how to proceed.

ALLERGY OR ILLNESS?

Allergies can be responsible for an extraordinary range of symptoms, but most of these can have alternative causes. How can you tell if your symptoms are part of an allergic condition?

COULD YOU BE SUFFERING FROM AN ALLERGY?

If the doctor cannot help you, ask yourself some basic questions:

► *Are your symptoms chronic or persistent? Do you have many, unrelated symptoms? These are classic markers of Type B allergies.*

► *Do you recall a time when you were free of symptoms? If your symptoms cleared up while you were away or on a different diet, it could be a useful clue about possible triggers.*

► *Have you noticed any regular correlations between your symptoms and certain situations or times? For instance, if they are worse in the morning, it may be that high levels of dust mite allergen or chemicals in your bedroom are to blame.*

Allergy or illness? This simple question goes to the heart of the controversy about allergy. The conventional medical view of allergies restricts the disorders caused by allergy to a few Type A conditions, such as asthma, hay fever and eczema. These conditions are well understood, and tend to be easy to diagnose, with characteristic symptoms of itching, wheezing, snuffles and runny eyes.

However, many other chronic illnesses may also be due to an allergy, although the link is harder to detect.

CHRONIC ILLNESS CAUSED BY ALLERGY

The chronic illnesses caused by allergy have three main features. First, the relationship between allergen and illness is often hidden. Second, patients are often allergic to more than one trigger, and may only react when triggers are encountered in combination. Third, patients usually suffer from multiple symptoms. So if you have migraine and irritable bowel syndrome, or rhinitis together with mood changes, you are very likely to be suffering from an allergy. Also, if your symptoms are worse during part of the menstrual cycle, or when you are under stress, allergies may be involved.

The 'hidden' nature of this sort of allergic reaction can prevent the patient from realising what is happening and so they continue to expose themselves to the triggers, leading to

DOCTOR KNOWS BEST
Have you been to see your doctor? You should check with your doctor if you are feeling ill. If he or she cannot identify the cause it might be worth considering allergies.

the development of chronic, often multiple symptoms. Some may be given a standard medical diagnosis, often more than one, but there may not be any abnormal physical findings or laboratory results.

Patients may also suffer multiple adverse drug reactions because this group of allergic patients is prone to develop side effects with drug treatments, particularly when many different drugs are tried.

WHAT SHOULD YOU DO IF YOU SUSPECT ALLERGY?

People who suspect that allergy is causing their symptoms should consult their GP before taking steps themselves to find out, since missing other diagnoses could be dangerous, delaying appropriate treatment.

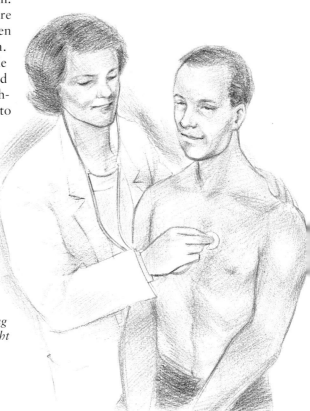

FACTORS THAT INDICATE ALLERGY

Allergy is more likely to be the cause of your symptoms if you react to medicines or there is a history of allergy in your family. Allergy is also suggested by a number of features which are characteristic of allergic conditions and help to distinguish them from other other illnesses. These features may be given a conventional interpretation, but can be indicative of allergy nonetheless.

IF YOUR SYMPTOMS...	EVEN IF...
... are variable	... you have not noticed a clear link between symptoms and changes in activity, place or time
... are multiple	... a standard diagnosis has been given for each
... respond to steroids	... your symptoms have been treated with antibiotics or other drugs
... differ in severity with activity, place or time	... they are also stress related, or get worse premenstrually

After ruling out serious diseases that could be responsible for the symptoms, investigations can be started to look for triggers that might be provoking an allergic reaction.

THE PROBLEM OF MULTIPLE SYMPTOMS

Most patients with Type B allergy complain of multiple symptoms. Detailed medical histories which look at how frequently a patient with Type B allergies has each symptom, show that most have five to ten symptoms, and 20 to 30 are not uncommon. Many are non-specific, for instance fatigue, sweating, insomnia, fluid retention, muscle pain and weight fluctuation. Others relate to asthma, eczema, rhinitis, migraine and irritable bowel syndrome, or even to well-recognised conditions such as arthritis or old injuries. When consulting the doctor, patients are usually very conscious of time constraints and concentrate on the major symptoms, leaving out the minor ones entirely; this may lead to a misdiagnosis.

Some doctors believe that patients with multiple symptoms (known as polysymptomatic) have 'somatisation syndrome' – they are developing physical symptoms because of psychological pain. Such doctors dispute that allergies can cause chronic, persistent Type B symptoms (see page 80).

PROOF ABOUT THE ROLE OF ALLERGIES

The medical histories of thousands of patients strongly suggest that many symptoms suffered by polysymptomatic patients are provoked by environmental factors, and that when these factors are removed or controlled the majority of the symptoms are relieved, either wholly or in part.

Those opposed to the allergy hypothesis argue that patients get better because of the extra attention they receive with this sort of therapy, or that the treatments simply have a placebo effect – patients believe that the treatment will work, and the psychological boost helps to counteract the psychological causes of the illness.

At the moment the anecdotal evidence can be interpreted either way, but there is a growing body of evidence from properly controlled studies that supports the theories of the environmentalists. If they are right, then there is little doubt that allergies and related problems like intolerances could be responsible for a wide range of illnesses.

HOW TO USE THIS SECTION

The directory of allergic disorders on the following pages covers the most common health problems linked with allergies. The disorders are grouped according to the body systems they affect.

► *Skin and bone disorders: skin inflammation, acne, soreness of mouth and lips and arthritis.*

► *Gastrointestinal disorders: including coeliac disease, colic, constipation, diarrhoea, irritable bowel syndrome and obesity.*

► *Nervous disorders: including insomnia, anxiety, mood disturbances, fatigue and headaches and migraine.*

► *Genitourinary disorders: including kidney and bladder problems, infertility and vaginal inflammation.*

► *Respiratory disorders: including sinusitis, ear problems, hay fever and asthma.*

Skin and Bone Disorders

An environmental approach to treating skin and bone disorders can help to clear up chronic problems that may not respond to conventional medical treatment. Using natural remedies to soothe symptoms can also reduce reliance on drugs.

SKIN INFLAMMATION

Urticaria (hives or nettle-rash) and eczema (dermatitis) are both types of skin inflammation that can be caused by allergies. Urticaria consists of an intensely itchy rash, made up of multiple weals. They usually have a red edge and a white centre, and last from a few hours to a day, but they may keep appearing in crops.

Eczema and dermatitis are terms that are often used interchangeably, and are characterised by dryness, flaking and cracking of the skin, accompanied by itching. Sometimes small bubbles form under the skin and may break open and weep.

Causes Urticaria may be provoked by physical factors such as cold, heat, exercise or pressure, but like eczema and dermatitis it can be caused by an allergic reaction, either by direct contact with an allergen, or through eating or inhaling one.

Treatment Urticaria is usually managed by antihistamines, although corticosteroids are sometimes needed. Standard medical treatment for eczema involves the use of moisturising agents, and corticosteroids, usually as a cream or lotion but sometimes taken orally. With young children it helps to stop them scratching (using mittens or swaddling), as scratching worsens the condition. However, in patients who react to something in skin cream – lanolin or preservative, for instance – even a corticosteroid cream can exacerbate eczema.

Supplements of zinc or evening primrose oil often help. The oil can be swallowed or rubbed on the skin. Natural remedies include calendula cream for dryness, chickweed ointment for itchiness, or camomile cream for both. Chinese medicine and homeopathy both have good track records in treating allergic skin problems, particularly eczema.

Neither conventional nor alternative treatments get to the root of the problem, however, and the best strategy is to avoid the triggers.

MAKING A SOOTHING CAMOMILE CREAM

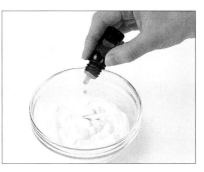 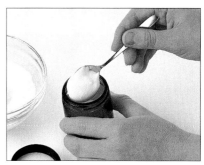

1 Mix 100 ml (3½ fl oz) of hypo-allergenic cream (available from a chemist) with 4-6 drops of essential oil of camomile. Blend thoroughly.

2 Spoon the mixture into a ster-ilised dark glass jar, to protect the contents from the light, and seal and label it with the date and contents.

ACNE

Acne is a chronic skin disorder characterised by spots mainly on the face and back.

Causes Acne is caused by inflammation of the hair follicles and the sebaceous glands in the skin. It is associated with puberty, greasy skin and the use of skin products which block the ducts. Allergic triggers can include contact with many of the allergens that cause eczema, and cosmetics, especially oil-based ones, are also common triggers. Food triggers can also cause acne.

Treatment Most commonly acne is treated with applications which unblock the pores and remove sebum. Exposure to ultraviolet and sunlight may help and oral antibiotics are also prescribed, though these may have side effects. Severe cases may be treated with retinoid drugs. A naturopathic approach would include drinking at least eight glasses of water a day and eating from five to eight servings of fresh fruit and vegetables a day.

SPOT TREATMENT
Herbalists may prescribe infusions (teas) of dandelion, nettle and burdock for acne treatment. These herbs are thought to remove toxins and cleanse the blood.

Nettle   Burdock   Dandelion

PREVENTION

▶ You should avoid putting oil on your face, including oil-based cosmetics and lotions. Drugs or foods may be contributing: you may need to try an elimination diet.

▶ Diet can help to control and prevent acne. Naturopaths recommend reducing your intake of dairy products, nuts, citrus fruit, sugar, white bread, red meat, caffeine and alcohol. Useful dietary supplements include zinc, taken at night apart from other nutrients, and vitamins A, B and C. Pregnant women or those planning a pregnancy, should not take more than 1200 mcg (4000 IU) of vitamin A a day.

SORE MOUTH AND LIPS

Marked swelling of the mouth and lips can be a sign of angio-oedema. If it involves the tongue or throat it could be dangerous – seek medical attention immediately.

Soreness of the mouth and lips can be due to mouth ulcers, and also to cold sores caused by the herpes simplex virus, which can affect the lips and face. Cracks at the corners of the mouth (angular stomatitis) can also be painful. However, in many patients who complain of sore or burning mouth or lips there is nothing abnormal to be seen, even when the symptoms are so bad that patients cannot tolerate eating anything at all hot or spicy.

Causes Mouth ulcers can be caused by deficiencies of iron or vitamin B in the diet, or by problems with dentures, particularly in the elderly. They can also be caused by allergic reactions to fillings. Where there is no obvious cause, hidden food allergies are often to blame. Cold sores are caused by the herpes simplex virus, but the virus may be dormant until triggered by ill health, stress or allergic illness.

Treatment Medication can be given to alleviate symptoms, but may not be much help. Antiviral creams such as acyclovir can prevent cold sores if used as soon as the warning tingling of an imminent attack is noticed. Herbal remedies may help relieve ulcers: make a soothing mouthwash by mixing a couple of drops each of geranium and lavender oil in a tumbler of water. A cooled infusion of liquorice combined with extract of red sage makes a mildly antiseptic mouthwash.

PREVENTION

▶ Ulcers and sores, and cases where there is discomfort with no apparent physical damage, will often respond to an elimination diet or avoidance of common chemical triggers (which may include commercial toothpastes or mouthwashes).

▶ Naturopaths suggest avoiding foods rich in arginine – such as nuts, chocolate, peas, cereals and garlic – and increasing intake of fish, cheese, brewer's yeast and yoghurt. Recovery can be quick, if all triggers are avoided, but may take up to four weeks.

LIP SERVICE
Geranium oil, diluted in sweet almond oil, can be rubbed in as an aromatherapy treatment for sore mouth and lips.

ARTHRITIS

Arthritis is an inflammatory condition which can affect any joint in the body, including those in the spine. It usually starts in the lining of the joint, the synovial membrane, but can spread to cartilage and bone. It causes symptoms of pain, swelling, stiffness and limited movement. In severe cases, it may lead to long term joint damage and deformity.

Causes There are numerous types of arthritis, some due to infections, some due to metabolic disorders and many of unknown origin. The commonest two types of arthritis are rheumatoid arthritis and osteoarthritis. In osteoarthritis normal wear and tear is thought to be a major cause. Rheumatoid arthritis is almost certainly due to an auto-immune response. Some allergists believe that allergic reactions – in particular hidden food allergies – may be involved in these and other types of arthritis, a view that is gaining currency as studies

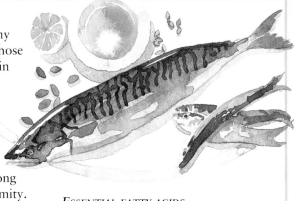

ESSENTIAL FATTY ACIDS
You can get essential fatty acids from a variety of sources, including evening primrose oil supplements, oily fish, such as mackerel or sardines, pumpkin seeds, or oil from linseed (also known as flax).

increasingly show that changing eating habits can reduce the severity of arthritis.

Treatment Conventional treatments may include analgesics, non-steroidal anti-inflammatory drugs and corticosteroids. These drugs only treat symptoms, not root causes, and corticosteroids suppress the immune system, which can cause side effects.

ARTHRITIS AND JOINTS

Joints like the hip joint shown below are where two bones articulate against one another. To lubricate and cushion the joint, it is sealed in a capsule lined with synovial membrane and filled with synovial fluid. The articulating surfaces of the bone are covered in smooth, protective, friction-reducing cartilage.

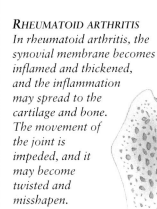

RHEUMATOID ARTHRITIS
In rheumatoid arthritis, the synovial membrane becomes inflamed and thickened, and the inflammation may spread to the cartilage and bone. The movement of the joint is impeded, and it may become twisted and misshapen.

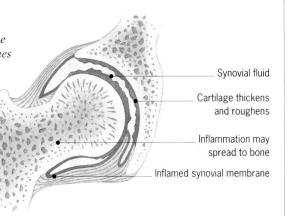

Synovial fluid

Cartilage thickens and roughens

Inflammation may spread to bone

Inflamed synovial membrane

Gastrointestinal Disorders

Although food allergies and intolerances can cause problems for almost every system of the body, they are particularly associated with digestive and gut disorders. These cause discomfort and pain and can also affect nutrient absorption and general health.

COELIAC DISEASE

Coeliac disease is a chronic condition involving the small bowel (the upper intestine). It is characterised by poor absorption of nutrients, diarrhoea, weight loss, mouth ulcers and sometimes a characteristic skin lesion (dermatitis herpetiformis).

Causes This condition is caused by sensitivity to gluten which is contained in wheat, barley and rye and in smaller quantities in oats and buckwheat. Even small doses of gluten can damage the intestinal wall in coeliac sufferers. Coeliac disease usually starts in childhood but can occur at any age. Though not precisely an allergy, coeliac disease is caused by an immunological reaction.

Treatment There is no medication that will make any specific improvement in this condition. Strict avoidance of gluten will normally produce complete relief of symptoms, and most sufferers can use rice or corn as substitutes for other grains. Vitamin B complex supplements may help. Ensure optimum levels of intestinal bacteria by taking bacterial supplements.

PREVENTION

▶ Coeliac problems can generally be prevented by strictly avoiding gluten (highest levels are found in wheat, barley, rye and oats).

▶ Some coeliacs also need to cut out other common trigger foods such as eggs or milk.

Herbs such as peppermint and ginger are said to aid digestive function and soothe the sensitive intestinal walls. Seek advice from a registered medical herbalist or naturopath.

COLIC

Also known as 'three month colic', this condition is caused by spasm of the bowel producing severe pain that causes the child to cry a great deal. It may be associated with vomiting and diarrhoea and other allergic conditions such as eczema.

DILL SEEDS
The seeds of the dill weed can be used to make a soothing infusion for colicky babies.

Causes The most common cause is milk allergy which occurs most frequently in bottle-fed babies but can also occur in breast-fed babies due to the mother passing on allergens that she has eaten.

Treatment Drugs can be used to reduce the pain and quiet the child. Feeding your baby a spoonful of fennel, dill seed or camomile infusion may also help to relieve pain. To make an infusion, pour 1 cup of boiled water over a teaspoon of dried herb (or half a teaspoon of crushed dill seed), leave for 5 minutes, strain off and allow to cool.

PREVENTION

▶ Bottle-fed children with colic may be helped by switching to either a soya-based formula or a hypo-allergenic milk product.

▶ Breastfeeding mothers might cut cow's milk out of their own diets, and perhaps other common culprit foods. If you are avoiding milk make sure you take a calcium supplement.

▶ If your baby has started mixed feeding, cut out wheat and juices and use a single food at each meal, until the culprit(s) is identified.

CONSTIPATION

Frequency of bowel movement varies widely between individuals, but if you also have hard, dry stools or difficulty in passing stools this is clear evidence of constipation.

Causes The major causes of constipation are too little exercise and eating too little fibre, but other causes can range from depression, to irritable bowel syndrome, to cancer. Constipation can be caused by allergies, especially if it alternates with periods of diarrhoea, and occurs together with other symptoms such as abdominal bloating or wind.

Treatment A high fibre diet, an increase in exercise and ensuring a fluid intake of at least two litres (three to four pints) a day if possible are the most effective steps. However, some people report that their symptoms become worse if they take bran, which suggests a wheat allergy. Avoiding wheat products and using a different product may be effective. If there is no improvement then you should check with a doctor to exclude serious organic causes such as cancer. Over-the-counter medications should be restricted to short-term use only, and the same applies to laxative herbal remedies like infusions of fenugreek, linseed (flax seed) or vervain.

STOMACH MASSAGE
Massaging your lower abdomen may help to relieve the symptoms of constipation. Rhythmically stroke the abdomen, using undulating pressure in a triangle around the navel.

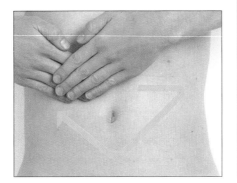

PREVENTION

▶ Eating a healthy diet which is high in fresh fruit, vegetables and fibre is the most important step in preventing constipation, but a significant number of people with constipation have evidence of food intolerance or allergy, and do not improve until the food or foods concerned are detected and avoided; trigger foods are commonly multiple.

▶ In children, milk products are the most common triggers, while cereals are the more common contributing factor in adults.

▶ A wide range of other foods may provoke constipation – even fruit, which is often eaten to increase the fibre content of the diet. If fruit makes the condition worse, avoid it and try drinking more water, eating fibrous foods that you can tolerate and perhaps using supplements to compensate for missing nutrients.

DIARRHOEA

Diarrhoea is a common condition, usually associated with three or more loose motions a day, but in extreme cases up to 30 a day. The motions are usually runny and may contain undigested food, mucus or blood.

Causes There are many causes of diarrhoea, the commonest being infections and irritable bowel syndrome (see page 147). Other causes include stress and enzyme deficiencies, such as lactose intolerance. If diarrhoea persists serious causes must be eliminated, especially the chronic inflammatory diseases, Crohn's disease and ulcerative colitis. Diarrhoea is also a very common symptom of hidden food allergy, which may even play a role in causing these other diseases.

Treatment Drug treatments such as loperamide can be used to control diarrhoea in the short-term. Severe diarrhoea causes upsets in the balance of salts in the blood; rehydration salts are available from pharmacists, and should be taken according to the instructions. Aromatherapy with lavender, camomile, juniper or sandalwood essential oils is said to relieve stress – add 6 to 8 drops of one of these to your bath, or inhale the vapours from a bowl of steaming water. Other relaxing therapies such as deep breathing may help in the case of stress-induced diarrhoea. Homeopaths may recommend *Arsenicum* or *Carbo veg.*

PREVENTION

▶ Elimination diets to identify triggers, with subsequent avoidance of the foods causing the problems, are the most effective prevention in cases where diarrhoea is caused by hidden food allergy or irritable bowel syndrome. When other conditions are responsible, dietary measures may not be sufficient, and they may require medical supervision.

TASTY TREATMENT
A teaspoon of honey with one drop each of peppermint and cypress oil, taken every two hours, may help to control diarrhoea.

IRRITABLE BOWEL SYNDROME

Irritable bowel syndrome (IBS) is now very common, especially in women – some estimates have suggested that at least half of women of reproductive age may have IBS. The diagnosis is usually made after other diseases have been excluded.

Typical symptoms are recurrent abdominal pain associated with bloating, wind, constipation and diarrhoea, which often alternate. In women symptoms are often worse just before menstruation.

Causes The most common cause is Type B food allergy and this responds well to the detection and avoidance of food triggers. The next most common cause is an imbalance in the gut micro-organisms, usually the overgrowth of fungi, which is exacerbated by diets that include a lot of refined carbohydrates (sugars and white flours). The third cause is lactose intolerance; this can

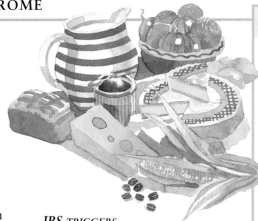

IBS TRIGGERS
The main culprits tend to be wheat or corn, milk products, tea, coffee, onions, potatoes and citrus fruit.

sometimes be difficult to distinguish from allergy to milk, but there are tests to differentiate. All these conditions are more likely to occur after gut infections and the use of antibiotics.

Treatment It is important to exclude serious non-allergic causes which can have similar symptoms.

PREVENTION

▶ Detection and avoidance of foods that provoke symptoms is usually so successful that patients no longer need medication or a particularly high fibre diet.

▶ Any food may be involved – sufferers should be aware that there are often several triggers acting in combination.

▶ Patients should eat a good diet, reduce stress levels and avoid antibiotics as far as possible.

The traditional medical treatment is a high fibre diet, drugs, avoidance of caffeine and stress reduction. For patients who do not improve, an elimination diet should be the next step – nearly all patients get partial or complete relief if they can detect and avoid their triggers. Anti-yeast treatment may be necessary for fungal overgrowth.

OBESITY

Obesity is a major problem in the West, where calorie consumption is high and general activity levels are decreasing. A recent survey by the National Centre for Disease Prevention in the US estimated that 35 per cent of Americans are 'dangerously overweight' – roughly 70 million people. In the UK the government estimates that more than 14 per cent of adults are obese.

Causes Obesity can be caused by hidden food allergy, which can result in fluid retention and cravings. Also,

the most common allergenic foods – wheat, eggs and milk – are often ingredients of high calorie foods.

Treatment To control obesity it is necessary to reduce calorie intake and increase activity levels. If these measures are tried properly and do not succeed, you could try an elimination diet, particularly if you also have other symptoms. Weigh yourself morning and night during the challenge period and avoid any foods that cause a weight gain of more than 1 kg (2 lb) over the day.

PREVENTION

▶ The best way to prevent obesity is to encourage healthy eating habits from childhood, avoiding sweets, refined foods and sugary drinks. Detecting hidden food allergies in diet-resistant obesity can make a significant contribution.

▶ Exposure to non-tolerated chemicals can also cause fluid retention and food craving, so you should consider possible sources of exposure to chemicals.

CHAIN OF FOOD
Allergies can act to increase weight in several ways, and these mechanisms may interact to make each other worse.

Hidden food allergy causes cravings for allergenic food → Cravings cause binging on high-calorie food triggers → Fluid retention results and general health deteriorates → Sufferer unwell and takes less exercise; metabolic rate falls, so calories not burnt

Nervous Disorders

The role of allergies in psychological disturbances and problems involving the central nervous system is controversial and the subject of much debate, but dietary and environmental measures are known to be effective in relieving nervous disorders.

INSOMNIA

The term insomnia is something of a catch-all term. It covers a variety of sleep-related problems, including difficulty in getting to sleep, waking early, disturbed sleep (waking frequently during the night), and not feeling rested in the morning.

Causes Anything which causes stress, tension, anxiety or physical discomfort can lead to insomnia. Too much caffeine is a common cause, as is eating late at night.

   Environmental causes are not uncommon. Hidden food allergies are known to produce insomnia, especially allergies to food additives and contaminants which also provoke hyperactivity. Exposure to volatile chemicals, particularly those from furniture and building materials (see Chapter 3) may also be to blame. House dust mite allergens, which may be at their highest concentration in the bedroom, can be a causative agent. Pollens and moulds are less likely to be directly responsible, but may have an indirect effect by causing nasal obstruction or wheezing.

Treatment The standard treatment for insomnia is a healthy diet of fresh foods, avoiding those containing additives or a lot of sugar, and cutting out drinks containing caffeine. Take regular meals, don't eat after seven at night, have regular exercise, and practise relaxation techniques. Ideally sedatives should not be used for more than a few days at a time.

   There are many complementary remedies for insomnia. They include a few drops of lavender oil on your pillow at night, rosemary oil baths, mustard foot baths and several traditional Chinese medicines. Homeopaths recommend *Coffea* to counteract mental restlessness.

   A naturopathic treatment for insomnia is to wash your legs before going to bed, and then try a relaxation routine. A simple technique you can practise in bed is progressive muscle relaxation. Get settled comfortably in bed and breathe deeply and steadily. Starting at your toes, focus on a group of muscles, tense them, and then relax them, concentrating on the feelings this causes. From the feet, work up through your legs, arms, abdomen, chest, back, neck and, finally, face.

COOL AND RELAXING
Bathe your feet and legs in cold water for 2 to 3 minutes, then dry them carefully and lie on your bed.

PREVENTION

▶ Reduce exposure to volatile chemicals and other airborne triggers in the house and at work. Try an elimination diet to identify and avoid food triggers.

▶ Try to reduce stress and tension. Beating your allergies can help with this, by increasing your tolerance for stress, and making you healthier and therefore happier.

▶ Sleep disturbance caused by nasal obstruction may need surgery, but a simple change in sleeping position could be equally effective.

ANXIETY

Anxiety is a normal emotional response to stress, but it may also occur when there is no reason to be anxious. It is often accompanied by symptoms like shortness of breath, hyperventilation, panic attacks, dizziness and sweating.

Causes Anxiety attacks are associated with some psychological conditions, with premenstrual tension and with thyroid problems.

They are more likely to occur in people who consume an excessive amount of caffeine.

Food intolerance and allergy can also cause anxiety attacks which occur for no obvious reason – but sometimes this only happens premenstrually or during periods of stress. Patients who suffer from multiple chemical sensitivity can have anxiety attacks as a result of exposure to chemicals.

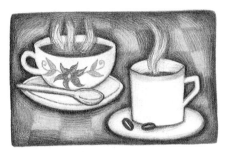

CUT DOWN ON YOUR CAFFEINE
Caffeine intake should be reduced to a daily maximum of 50 mg (roughly one cup of tea or half a cup of coffee).

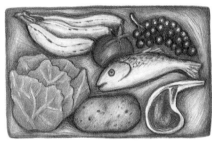

BOOST YOUR FRESH FOODS
Eating more fruit, vegetables, fish and meat will provide beneficial B vitamins, magnesium and other minerals.

Treatment Counselling, reducing stress and the controlled use of tranquillisers and antidepressants are the usual ways of dealing with the symptoms. Naturopaths advocate nutritional therapy including vitamin B complex and magnesium.

Try to reduce your exposure to chemicals, and identify any food allergies using the Stone Age Diet. Be prepared for panic attacks when doing food challenges – make sure you have help and support on hand.

MOOD DISTURBANCES

Depression, aggression, anxiety, irritability and, particularly in children, hyperactivity, have all been linked with allergies. Allergic reactions may even be a factor in causing criminal behaviour.

Causes A variety of factors affect mood. Mood changes are usually attributed to genetic make-up, psychological factors or stress, but allergic reactions to environmental factors and foods are a frequent cause. Foods and food additives are commonly responsible for hyperactivity in children and irritability in adults. In young children milk, wheat or juice are the leading culprits. In older children colourings and other additives are the most common causes but sugars, milk products and other foods may

also be responsible. In older patients reactions to alcohol, cigarette smoke, coffee and fizzy drinks containing additives are common causes of irritability. Some cases of depression have been shown to be due to sensitivity to wheat and dairy products but allergy to any food can be responsible. Deficiencies of the B vitamins may also cause mental problems, including depression, as may chemical odours – air fresheners are a common culprit.

Treatment Although there are many drugs for their treatment, mood disturbances can be very difficult to control satisfactorily. Disturbances are often transient, lasting only a few hours, making drug control difficult without producing unacceptable side effects. In the US, powerful drugs are

widely used to treat hyperactive children with variable success and uncertain side effects. If possible, it is better to identify the triggers and avoid exposure. Supplements of B vitamins and minerals such as magnesium and zinc can be helpful.

FATIGUE

Fatigue refers to excessive tiredness that is out of proportion to a person's level of activity or exercise. In chronic fatigue syndrome (CFS, also referred to as ME) fatigue is usually unrelieved by rest, worse in the morning showing gradual improvement during the day, but getting worse after minimal exertion. Severe exertion can leave the patient bedridden for days.

Causes Fatigue is extremely common, and is a symptom of many diseases. In one survey in the US, 50 per cent of patients admitted to hospital gave fatigue as one of their major symptoms. Fatigue commonly accompanies hay fever and other allergic reactions caused by airborne allergens, and chemicals such as formaldehyde or toluene.

Hidden food allergy (particularly, but not only, to milk products) and environmental allergies are often associated with fatigue. Disturbed sleep and insomnia, directly or indirectly caused by allergic reactions, can cause tiredness and lethargy.

Chronic fatigue syndrome is now recognised as a definite and very disabling illness, which is still not fully understood. In the early stages it is important to rest; later, muscles must be gently exercised, increasing the exercise gradually but being careful not to worsen symptoms. Patients with CFS who also have other symptoms are often helped by investigation for allergies.

Treatment There is no specific drug treatment for fatigue. Tranquillisers often make symptoms worse; antidepressants can be helpful especially when there is also depression. Fatigue often disappears when the allergic causes are identified. Supplements of essential fatty acids, magnesium and vitamin B_{12} can be useful. Chinese energy tonics containing ginseng may help. Herbs like passionflower are recommended for a good night's sleep, and acupressure may help to boost energy levels.

WHEN AND WHERE?
Think about foods and environments which seem to affect your fatigue. You might identify times and places where it is worse and this could give you clues about the triggers which may be causing your problem.

PREVENTION

▶ Fatigue may be associated with low blood sugar levels which can follow a sugar boost, so avoid sweets. Have savoury snacks, such as water biscuits, nuts, seeds, and cheese on rice crackers, midway between the three main meals of the day.

▶ Fatigue is also common in cases of allergy and intolerance, so if no obvious physical cause is found, a food history, followed by an elimination diet is the next step. Milk products are high on the list of foods that can cause fatigue but grains, tea, coffee and other foods can also be triggers.

▶ At the same time an environmental cleanup to reduce exposure to inhalant allergens and chemicals should be undertaken both at home and at work. Improvement in the condition during a holiday away from home and work would suggest an environmental cause, usually related to inhalant allergens or chemicals but maybe to a food which was not eaten while abroad.

TENSION AND FATIGUE

Fatigue sufferers often find that their tiredness is accompanied by a constant state of tension, leaving them feeling both tense and exhausted. This combination of symptoms is found in both adults and children, where it can form part of the constellation of symptoms involved in hyperactivity (see page 136). Sufferers often exhibit 'allergic shiners' – dark circles under their eyes – which can act as a key marker for allergic fatigue.

HEADACHES AND MIGRAINE

Many terms are used to describe headaches – constant, throbbing, aching, stabbing. They often affect both sides of the head, and may spread down into the neck or shoulders. Migraine is a complex of symptoms of which headache is just one. Other symptoms include disturbed vision, hunger, thirst, hypersensitivity to light, noise and movement, and very often nausea and vomiting. Migraine can last for anything from a few hours to two or three days, and is commonly followed by fatigue and hypersensitivity to stimuli. In children it is associated with abdominal pain, with the headache element becoming dominant as the child gets older.

Causes Headaches can accompany a lot of different illnesses, such as infections, stress, muscle spasm, eye or ear problems, but most headaches are not accompanied by any demonstrable illness; some have environmental causes. Migraine is rarely associated with an obvious disease and is usually provoked by environmental factors.

Treatment When treatable illnesses have been excluded as a cause, treatment usually concentrates on relieving symptoms using painkillers and non-steroidal anti-inflammatory drugs. A variety of drugs may be used for migraine, include anti-vomiting drugs and, in severe cases, strong analgesics by injection.

Yoga, t'ai chi and the Alexander technique are all useful for relieving stress and helping with headaches. Feverfew is a well-established herbal remedy for migraine, and reflexology is often used to relieve pain and other symptoms. Many people have found osteopathy and acupuncture beneficial in relieving headaches.

PREVENTION

▶ The role of hidden food allergy in migraine has been firmly established in trials involving both adults and children. In some cases simple changes may be sufficient, such as not skipping a meal, or avoiding caffeine. In most other cases a diet such as the Stone Age Diet (see page 84) may be enough to find the culprits.

▶ In the most severe cases diets may need to be undertaken with medical supervision because withdrawal reactions and the reactions to food challenges can be severe.

▶ Steps should also be taken to reduce exposure to chemicals and airborne allergens.

▶ Avoiding trigger foods is usually just as effective with other sorts of headache as it is with migraine.

A SIMPLE YOGA POSE FOR HEADACHE RELIEF

Yoga is an excellent therapy for sufferers of migraines and headaches, particularly as it relieves muscular tension, often a cause of headaches. Shown below is a move called a supine twist, with an added element, a pad between your shoulder blades – you can use a tightly folded sock – which customises the pose for headache relief.

1 *Lie on your back with the folded sock underneath your spine, between your shoulder blades. Slowly bring your knees up, and put your right arm behind your thighs, hugging your knees to your chest. Let your left arm lie at your side. Roll your head to the left, keeping your chin tucked in.*

2 *Move your left arm so that it is at right angles to your body. Exhale, and, keeping your head turned to the left and your shoulders on the ground, roll your legs and hips to the right. Breathe in and out and bring your arms and legs back to the centre. Repeat to the reverse side.*

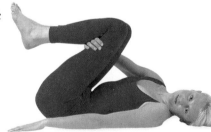

HEADACHE AND MIGRAINE TRIGGERS

Alcohol, smoking and the contraceptive pill contribute to both headaches and migraine; food probably plays a part in at least 60 per cent of cases. Chemicals and inhalant allergens can also be responsible. Foods recognised as triggers of migraine include coffee, chocolate, cheese, bananas, red wine and citrus fruit but any hidden food allergy can cause migraine, as can sensitivity to pollens, house dust mite allergens, animals and volatile chemicals. Headaches may also be caused by dental work or by physical problems which have misaligned the jaw or the neck.

Genitourinary Disorders

Problems such as infertility and kidney disease fall outside the range of disorders normally attributed to allergies. However, in some cases, uncovering and avoiding allergic triggers can help to resolve apparently intractable conditions.

KIDNEY AND BLADDER PROBLEMS

Allergic reactions can cause serious kidney problems including fluid retention, blood or protein in the urine, and severe pain. Bladder symptoms may be caused by urinary infection but the same symptoms – lower abdominal pain and difficulties with passing urine (frequency, pain and urgency) – can be caused by allergic reactions. In children allergies can cause bed-wetting, and in the elderly a worsening of stress incontinence. Kidney problems may be very serious, so always report them to your doctor.

Causes The kidneys and bladder are the major excretory system of the body, which means that many allergenic substances pass through them. Bladder irritation may also be caused by toiletries used around the genitals, fabrics used in underwear and washing powders and fabric conditioners. Foods are by far the most common cause of allergic bladder symptoms in children, especially grains and fruits, but reactions to medication may also cause bladder symptoms.

Treatment One measure to relieve symptoms is to increase fluid intake to at least 2 litres (3 to 4 pints) of fluid a day. This can help to wash the causes of irritation away, whether they are bacteria or allergens. Another is to make your urine more alkaline by eating more alkaline foods (vegetables and fruit, but not citrus fruit) and reducing protein and cereal intake.

Homeopathic remedies like *Nux vomica* and *Apis mel* may help to relieve the urge to urinate and pain in the lower abdomen.

HELP FOR YOUR WATERWORKS
Infusions (essentially herbal teas) of couch grass, marshmallow, parsley and yarrow can soothe urinary problems.

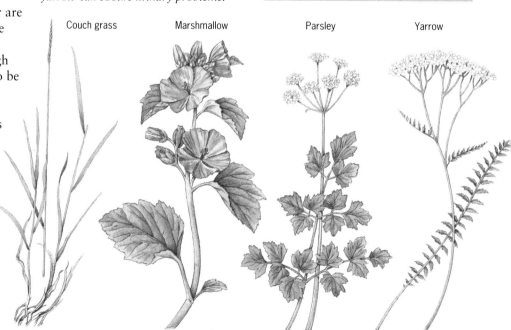

Couch grass · Marshmallow · Parsley · Yarrow

INFERTILITY

Infertility is defined as the inability of a couple to conceive after trying for a child for at least a year, although the time interval is arbitrary. Some doctors insist on a longer time before starting investigations, depending on the age of the couple.

Causes The last 40 years have seen a significant reduction in sperm count in men. The reason for this is not yet clearly established, but increased use of hormones, the effect of chemicals which mimic hormones and exposure to pesticides are all suspected causes. A number of conditions can contribute to infertility in women, ranging from being underweight to infections which can block the Fallopian tubes. Drinking, smoking and nutritional deficiencies damage the fertility of both sexes.

Allergy can play a part in some cases, but allergic infertility can be reversed if investigations identify sensitivities to foods, inhalants or chemicals (or to a combination of them) and appropriate avoidance measures are taken. In one patient a sensitivity to milk was shown to inhibit ovulation. In rare cases, women become allergic to their partner's semen so the immune system attacks and destroys sperm.

Treatment The first step is normally to exclude infection and treat any other possible cause. If this is unsuccessful, hormonal therapy or various fertility treatments (such as artificial insemination or IVF) may be used. Supplements to rectify nutritional deficiencies and avoiding exposure to environmental allergens can be very successful in some patients. Acupuncture may also be able to help. Herbal medicines may not have been tested for safety of use during pregnancy.

ALLERGY AND INFERTILITY
An allergist can help you to identify chemicals and foods from your environment that could be causing or contributing to infertility. Avoiding them could be the best therapy.

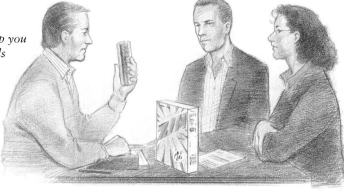

PREVENTION

▶ Improving diet, including supplements of vitamins, zinc, magnesium and selenium, and maintaining good general health and fitness, together with not smoking are important for both men and women.

▶ Keeping the testicles cool by avoiding tight trousers and hot baths can help men to keep up their sperm counts.

▶ Maintaining a healthy body weight and a balanced diet is essential for women looking to improve their fertility and have healthy babies.

VAGINAL INFLAMMATION

Vaginal inflammation (vaginitis) is associated with soreness, itching and discharge. It varies in severity from a slight nuisance to a debilitating handicap, with symptoms of cystitis and severe pain making sexual intercourse impossible.

Causes The commonest cause is probably infection, particularly thrush, but vaginitis can also be caused by contact allergies to rubber, artificial fibres, dyes and finishes in fabrics, toiletries and medications of any sort. Allergies to contraceptives are becoming more common, particularly latex allergy to diaphragms or condoms. Women can also become sensitised to their partner's seminal fluid. Food, chemical and inhalant reactions can all cause reactions in the vagina.

Treatment Infectious causes must be treated appropriately, but topical medication should be used with care because sensitisation can easily occur. Natural yoghurt and a diet low in sugars and refined starch are effective natural treatments for thrush, but you should seek medical advice for any vaginal inflammation.

PREVENTION

▶ Identifying and avoiding irritants and allergens is essential. Consider everything that comes into contact with your perineum, including clothes and the detergents they are washed in.

▶ Hidden food allergy should be considered, and inhalant allergens, especially if vaginitis is seasonal.

A medical herbalist may prescribe soothing pessaries or douches to correct any imbalances in the vaginal secretions.

Respiratory Disorders

This group includes some of the classic allergic disorders, such as hay fever and asthma. Disorders of the ears and sinuses also fall under this heading as they are areas related to the respiratory tract and involve irritation of mucous membranes.

HAY FEVER AND RHINITIS

Rhinitis symptoms typically involve the nose (itching, runny nose and sneezing, or a congested, blocked nose) and may be accompanied by eye symptoms (itching, sensitivity to bright lights and discharge). Hay fever is a seasonal allergic rhinitis which most often occurs during the summer months, usually during the grass pollen season, but it can occur throughout most of the year. In hay fever the palate and throat may also itch, and the patient feels unwell, with headaches and fatigue.

Causes Hay fever during May and June is usually caused by exposure to grass pollen, but at other times it can be due to tree and other pollens, or to seasonal mould spores. Perennial rhinitis, where symptoms persist all year round, is caused by house dust mite droppings, pet hairs, mould spores and chemical fumes, or by hidden food allergy.

Treatment In mild cases, treatment with nasal decongestants and antihistamines is usually sufficient, but steroid sprays, injections and tablets may be used. Desensitisation can be effective. Essential oil of lavender can soothe nasal symptoms. Homeopathic remedies like *Gelsemium* and *Arsenicum album* are said to help with blocked and runny noses, sore eyes and sneezing. Splashing the face and sinus areas with warm water for 2 minutes then cold water for 1 minute, can provide some relief.

PREVENTION

▶ In 50 per cent of perennial rhinitis cases, inhaled allergens are involved, possibly in combination with food allergy, which is the main cause in most of the rest.

▶ Milk is a leading trigger of rhinitis. Both environmental measures and an elimination diet are often needed, but of the two detection and avoidance of trigger foods is more likely to give dramatic improvement; for some people just excluding all milk products may be sufficient.

FIRST LINE OF DEFENCE
For short-term relief hay fever sufferers can use decongestants and antihistamines.

SINUSITIS

If the mucous membranes lining the sinuses become inflamed, the openings can get blocked causing a build-up of mucus. This may result in pressure and pain, possibly leading to infection (acute sinusitis).

Causes Sinusitis can be caused by bacterial infections of the membranes lining the sinuses, but allergic rhinitis is often to blame.

Treatment Antihistamines and decongestants may give short-term relief but they can exacerbate symptoms in the long run. Naturopaths recommend natural decongestants like fenugreek, or simple heat or steam, and natural antihistamines like vitamin C. These may be as effective as conventional medication, without the side effects. Sponging the face with water,

PREVENTION

▶ Most cases of rhinitis-induced sinusitis respond to the detection and avoidance of environmental triggers.

alternating 2 minutes with hot water and 1 minute with cold, can provide relief. Antibiotics may be needed for acute sinusitis.

ASTHMA

In asthma the airways in the lungs are hyper-reactive and can go into spasm, causing shortness of breath and wheezing as they become constricted and mucus is secreted. The condition is very common: in the last 20 years the incidence has rocketed, especially amongst children – about 3 million people are now affected in the UK, a number which looks set to rise.

> ### WARNING
> *Asthmatics should take great care when trying food challenges – even when they are investigating other conditions. Food challenges taken after avoiding a trigger for a week can cause unexpectedly severe reactions. Consult your doctor first.*

Causes The underlying cause of asthma is inflammation of the airways due to release of chemicals such as histamine. In the vast majority of asthmatics release is provoked by allergic reactions to one or more environmental allergens or foods, and if you look hard enough the cause or causes can almost always be found.

Treatment Asthma is treated with a variety of medications – primarily bronchodilators, disodium cromoglycate – mainly for children – and corticosteroids (see page 45). However, most of these medications are aimed at suppressing symptoms rather than attacking the cause of the problem. Drinking plenty of liquids, particularly hot liquids, can help to clear mucus from the airways. Learning to relax your breathing is also a major step in reducing the severity of attacks.

PREVENTION

▶ The best treatment for asthma is prevention – above all this means identifying and avoiding the triggers that cause your asthma. The majority of asthmatics can be helped by taking basic steps to avoid the most common environmental triggers and the most common food allergens (see Chapters 3 and 4).

▶ Other important factors in prevention are fitness, weight and nutrition. Fit people are better at extracting oxygen from the air they breathe; slim people have less weight around the diaphragm which makes it easier to breathe. Magnesium deficiency makes asthma worse and so a supplement of this mineral should be considered, as well as eating a diet high in fresh fruit and vegetables.

EAR PROBLEMS

Chronic glue ear, where the middle ear fills with fluid, is a common condition in young children, but is also found in adults. Inflammation of the inside of the ear is also a problem for both adults and children, and can lead to permanent hearing loss.

Causes The exact cause of glue ear is unknown. The common cold is often thought to be a cause in children, but the 'cold' may be evidence of allergy, not infection. Rhinitis, whatever the cause, leads to blocking of the Eustachian tube and a build-up of fluid in the ear. Ear inflammation is more likely when tonsillitis or sinusitis are also present, and these can be made worse by allergy.

Treatment Decongestants can be effective, but in severe cases small tubes (called grommets) are inserted through the ear drums to drain off fluid. Homeopaths suggest *Pulsatilla* to improve drainage and *Ferrum phos.* for earache.

EAR RELIEF
A hot water bottle wrapped in a towel and held over the ear may help to provide quick relief from pain.

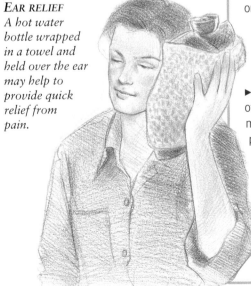

PREVENTION

▶ Over 80 per cent of children with glue ear have rhinitis and when the causes of rhinitis are found and eliminated, hearing improves and only a few require grommets. In many cases airborne allergens are to blame, but in at least 10 per cent of cases, glue ear is due to Type B allergies to foods.

▶ Milk is usually one trigger but other foods may also be involved. It may be enough to avoid milk products, but these must be cut out completely and children not drinking milk should probably take a calcium and magnesium supplement.

▶ Also, eat more vegetables and reduce sugars and additives in the diet.

GLOSSARY

Allergen: an *antigen* that causes an allergic reaction.

Angio-oedema: a reaction that causes swelling in the deeper layers of the skin, especially the face and lips.

Antibody: a protein molecule made by the body in response to a foreign molecule, or antigen. Antibodies are designed to recognise one specific antigen. They belong to a class of proteins called *immunoglobulins*.

Antigen: any substance that elicits an immune response.

Anaphylaxis: a generalised allergic reaction leading to shock and collapse. If not treated, anaphylaxis can be fatal.

Atopy: a general tendency to overproduce *IgE*, and thus be highly allergic. Allergic reactions like hay fever are manifestations of atopy.

Challenge: exposing the sufferer to a suspect substance (e.g. a food or scent) in order to see if it provokes a reaction.

Chronic: a long-term and/or recurring health condition.

Complement: a group of chemical messengers in the blood that play a part in inflammation and the activation of *phagocytes* and other immune cells.

Cytotoxicity: literally the killing of a cell, whether by another cell (e.g. a cytotoxic T-cell) or by a chemical.

Dander: tiny skin particles from animals or birds that can cause an allergy in susceptible individuals.

Dermatitis: a general term for skin inflammation, including *eczema*. Some dermatitis is allergic, but often the cause is unknown.

Desensitisation: a procedure to reduce an individual's sensitivity to an allergen. There are several different types. Also called immunotherapy.

Eczema: a skin condition where patches of skin become thickened, red and itchy and may erupt into blisters that weep and crust over.

Elimination diet: a diet used to identify the foods responsible for hidden food allergies. People limit their diets to foods least likely to cause problems until symptoms settle down.

Essential fatty acids (EFAs): components of fats and oils that play an essential part in metabolic processes but cannot be made in the body. They are important in cell walls, in nerves, and in some of the messengers in the immune system.

Evening primrose oil: oil from the seeds of the evening primrose plant. Contains the *essential fatty acid*, gammalinoleic acid (GLA), helpful in a number of allergies, including *eczema*.

Food intolerance: a term which can be used for all adverse reactions to foods not due to an obvious allergy, or just for those that are due to deficiencies in enzymes which interfere with the digestion or metabolism of food.

Gluten: gluten is the main protein in wheat, also found in rye, barley and oats to varying degrees, which must be avoided by sufferers of coeliac disease.

Hidden food allergy: a food allergy where the link between symptoms and ingesting a particular food is not obvious. For instance, symptoms may be vague, take a long time to come on, or affect parts of the body other than the gut.

Histamine: an important inflammatory chemical messenger. Stored in granules in mast cells and released when they degranulate.

IgE: a type of *immunoglobulin* responsible for immediate allergy. IgE is usually carried on the surface of mast cells.

Immune-mediated: caused by specific reactions of cells or molecules of the immune system. Allergies, for instance, are immune-mediated.

Immunoglobulin (Ig): another name for the *antibody* class of proteins.

Inflammation: in response to injury, allergy or infection, the tissues of the body become painful, hot, red and swollen. *Phagocytes* and other cells flow into the affected area to clean up and promote healing.

Lymphocytes: immune cells that react to foreign molecules, or antigens. They include B and T-cells.

Masked food allergy: another name for *hidden food allergy*, where the trigger is ingested frequently enough for the symptoms from one reaction to fade into the next set of symptoms.

Oedema: swelling caused by fluid retention. It can be caused by kidney disease or by a food allergy or intolerance.

Phagocytes: a group name for cells that destroy foreign cells, particles and molecules by engulfing and digesting them. Types of phagocyte include macrophages and polymorphs.

Placebo: an inactive treatment given in place of real treatment. In a double-blind trial, for instance, a subject may be given a sugar pill instead of a drug. When a placebo treatment provokes a change in symptoms, this is called a placebo effect.

Polysymptomatic: experiencing many, apparently unrelated symptoms.

Pseudoallergy: when mast cells or other elements of the allergic response are triggered directly by a chemical, and not by a normal allergic mechanism, the effects appear the same as an allergic reaction, but are said to be pseudoallergic.

Radio-allergosorbent (RAST) test: the name of a test used to detect levels of *IgE* antibody in a person's blood.

Somatisation: the expression of psychological problems through physical symptoms. A term used by some doctors to explain Type B symptoms, which they argue have no physical cause.

Tolerance induction: the process whereby the immune system is encouraged to become tolerant of an *allergen*. Artificial tolerance induction is the aim of *desensitisation*.

Topical: applied locally – a topical steroid is one inhaled or applied directly to the skin.

Toxin: a poisonous or harmful substance. Toxins may come from outside the body – from bacteria, wasp stings, plants or human activities (toxic chemicals). Toxins may also be produced by cells inside the body.

Urticaria (nettle rash/hives): a condition where the skin becomes very itchy with swollen red blotches known as weals.

INDEX

157

ACKNOWLEDGMENTS

Carroll & Brown Limited
would like to thank
British Society for Allergy,
   Environmental and Nutritional
   Medicine, Southampton
Dr Sheldon Cohen, Scientific Advisor,
   National Institute of Allergy and
   Infectious Disease
Sharon Freed
Green and White Ltd
IDIS World Medicines
Margaret Moss
Sara Turner

Editorial assistance
Denise Alexander
Angela Newton
Laura Price

Design assistance
Mercedes Morgan
Karen Sawyer
Jonathan Wainwright

DTP design
Elisa Merino

Photograph sources
Cover K.H. Kjeldsen/Science Photo
   Library
   8 National Library of
      Medicine/Science Photo Library
   9 Kimishige Ishizaka, MD
   10 (Top) Wellcome Institute
      Library, London
      (Bottom) Frank Spooner/Hajdih
      Bruno
   16 Courtesy of the National
      Library of Medicine Collection,
      National Institutes of Health,
      Bethesda, Maryland, USA
   19 Eddy Gray/Science Photo
      Library
   25 B. Wittich/Custom Medical
      Stock Photo/Science Photo
      Library
   27 Telegraph Colour Library
   29 Dr Kari Lounatmaa/Science
      Photo Library
   30 Lori Adamski Peek/Tony
      Stone Images
   32 BSIP, LECA/Science
      Photo Library
   38 Reference material courtesy of
      Vega Grieshaber GmbH & Co
   34 Prof Gunnar Johansson
   37 Manfred Kage/Science
      Photo Library
   42 Carroll & Brown
   43 K.H. Kjeldsen/Science
      Photo Library
   51 James Strachan/Tony
      Stone Images
   54 David Stewart/Tony
      Stone Images
   56 Mary Evans Picture Library
   58 Eye of Science/Science
      Photo Library
   59 (Left) CNRI/Science
      Photo Library
      (Centre) Dr Jeremy Burgess/
      Science Photo Library
      (Right) David Scharf/
      Science Photo Library
   63 Images Colour Library
   68 Carroll & Brown
   72 CNRI/Science Photo Library
   74 Zigy Kaluzny/Tony
      Stone Images
   80 Chris Priest & Mark
      Clark/Science Photo Library
   81 Labat, Jerrigan/Science
      Photo Library
   84 Rex Features
   88 Andrew Syred/
      Microscopix Photolibrary
   93 Simon Fraser/Science Photo
      Library
   96 M. Ashley/Anthony Blake
   98 John G. Egan, Dublin/
      Hutchison Library
   102 Eye of Science/Science
      Photo Library
   103 Andrew Syred/
      Science Photo Library
   104 Hutchison Library
   112 Corbis-Bettman
   114 Dr Jeremy Burgess/
      Science Photo Library
   116 Wellcome Institute
      Library, London
   120 (Top) Dale Durfee/Tony
      Stone Images
      (Bottom) Hutchison Library/
      Maurice Harvey
   124 (Top) David Parker/Science
      Photo Library
   125 Claude Nuridsany and Marie
      Perennou/Science Photo Library
   126 The Movie Store
   130 Ron Sutherland/Science
      Photo Library
   132 Angela Hampton/Family
      Life Pictures

Medical illustrators
Paul Williams
Sandie Hill

Illustrators
John Geary
Nicola Gregory
Bill Piggins
Pond and Giles
Josephine Sumner
Anthea Whitworth

Computer generated artwork
Mick Gillah
Mirashade Ltd

Photographic assistants
M-A Hugo
Mark Langridge
Alex Franklin

Hair and make-up
Kim Menzies
Jessamina Owens

Picture research
Sandra Schneider

Research
Denise Alexander
Steven Chong

Index
Nadia Silver